Art and Cure
Past, Present and Future

Eurico de Aguiar

Eurico de Aguiar

About the author

Eurico de Aguiar is medical doctor; Master in Clinical Microbiology.

To health professionals who, throughout this new coronavirus pandemic, have shown a high level of dedication and professionalism.

"Brutus is sick ... And is it good for your health to go out almost without clothes and to breathe in the humid dawn moods? Brutus is ill and leaves his comfortable bed to expose himself to the pernicious contagion of the night and defy the cold and addicted air that will further increase his evil?".

Julius Caesar, second act[1].

Eurico de Aguiar

Introduction

The primitive art of cure

The beginning

The Chinese art of healing

The Mesopotamian art of healing

The Egyptian art of healing

The Hebrew Art of Healing

The Indian art of healing

The Greek art of healing

The Alexandria School

The Roman art of healing

Sorano

Galen

The decline of Rome and the rise of religious civilizations

The decline in the importance of the art of healing

Art and heal and Christianity

Paulus of Aegina

The Arabs

The first universities

The strologia and diseases

Physiotherapy

Amerindians and diseases

The art of healing of the Aztecs, Mayans and Incas

Most important diseases in the Middle Ages:

Leprosy

Black Plague

The black death of the sea

Other medieval diseases

The empirical art of cure

Eurico de Aguiar

New philosophical ideas

The Renaissance

Andreas Vesalius

The anatomical amphitheaters

Girolamo Fracastoro

Paracelsus

Jean Fernel

Ambroise Paré

Johann Weyer

Fabrizio de Acquapendente

European transformations

Johannes Kepler

Newtonian mechanics

William Harvey

The first societies and scientific journals

Leewnhoek

The first statistics

Thomas Sydeham

Boerhaave

John Hunter

Morgagni

The art of healing in Brazil

The first medical books published in Brazil

Bernardino Ramazzini

The French revolution

The release of the mentally ill

The beginning of medical geography

Johann Peter Frank

The industrial revolution and health reform

Laennec

Semmelweis

The emergence of homeopathy

The beginning of homeopathy in Brazil

Mesmer and animal magnetism

Beginning of experimental research in physiology

Most important diseases until the end of the Modern Age:

Tuberculosis

Cholera

Eurico de Aguiar

Modern Art of cure

Nineteenth century philosophical ideas

Louis Pasteur

Charles Darwin

Claude Bernard

The death of pain

Rudolph Virchow

Robert Koch

The consequences of advances in bacteriology, physiology and pathology

Gregor Johann Mendel

The art of healing in Brazil in the 19th century

The creation of public health laboratories in Brazil

Joseph Lister

The beginning of scientific dentistry

Bilroth and experimental surgery

A new nursing

Natural medicine

The emergence of pediatrics

The last enemy of surgery falls

The beginning of diagnostic imaging

Harrison

Erlich

Marie Curie

Oswaldo Cruz

The vaccine revolt

Carlos Chagas

Juliano Moreira

The discovery of insulin

Fleming

Freud and the creation of psychoanalysis

The natural history of diseases

Medical education in the USA

Most important diseases in the early 20th century:

Yellow fever

The flu

Contemporary art of cure

Eurico de Aguiar

The discovery of the genetic code

New technologies and the evolution of health sciences

Ethics in scientific research

A glance at history

Most important diseases at the end of the 20th century:

Chronic non-communicable diseases

Acquired immunodeficiency syndrome

Dengue

Covid -19

Relics of the art of cure

Contraceptive prescription

Recipe to know the sex of children

Revenue against cold

Plants used by traditional Chinese medicine

Plants used by the Mesopotamians

Recipe against cough

Prescription to eliminate kidney stones

Treatment of pneumonia

About teaching surgery

About medical ethics

On the nature of things

On how to deal with frustrations

Ash Wednesday Sermon

Recipe for aromatic fumigation

Recommendations for health preservation

Recipes against sadness

The difference between the true and the false doctor

Remedy for monthly bowel movement

The wisdom of life

The truth and research

About experimental science

Beyond good and evil

How to treat nerve attack

How to prevent baldness

How to treat diabetes

How to treat epilepsy

How to treat insomnia

Eurico de Aguiar

Psychotherapy

Hysteria

Breastfeeding the newborn

How to treat obesity

The defense of homeopathy

How to prevent headache and migraine

On the choice of medicine

About the history of science

On the complexity of nature

About the art of life

Epilogue

Acknowledgments

Bibliography

INTRODUCTION

When starting a book like this it is prudent to remember the teachings of Prof. Fernando Novais, for whom texts like this are not made with certainty or categorical statements. According to him, "in History, there can never be a definitive work; all we can aspire to are approximations".[two]

There were several sources where I searched to reach the final text. I agree with the view of the importance of understanding the history of health sciences not as a progressive line connected by advances and discoveries, but as part of a process, where a set of factors act and are related to each other.[3]

The main reason that led me to write this book was the realization that most medical schools around the world, including Brazil, have underestimated the importance of knowledge of the history of medicine.

Eurico de Aguiar

It is only after years of experience that some doctors are concerned with reading about philosophy and other cultural disciplines. At this point, then, they are also interested in this fascinating adventure throughout the ages.

Philosophers like Plato and Aristotle were students of the health sciences. Philosophy influenced medicine to the point of Kurt Sprengel[4] having said that "philosophy is the mother of medicine". Conversely, science has influenced philosophy, as examples are psychoanalysis and neurophysiological studies of how the intellect operates.

Philosophy and science are based on the same basis as the human spirit, that is, thought. However, they are distinguished by the object of study. While science has as its object portions of reality, philosophy seeks to address itself as a whole, that is, philosophy would be a kind of universal science and its function would be not so much to solve puzzles, but to discover wonders, oscillating its greatest interest. between the "conception of the self" and the "conception of the universe"[5].

According to Hegel, "philosophy, in dealing with the true, has only to do with the eternally present. For philosophy, everything that belongs to the past is rescued, because the idea is always present and the spirit is immortal; there is no past or future for her, only an essential *now* "[6].

I also believe that the lack of better humanistic training has brought serious consequences to the way in which health sciences have developed.

The repercussions of a mistaken view of health are reflected, in society, by the belief that the medical act is more important than the health policy actions to improve the population's quality of life.

On the other hand, it also negatively affects the doctor-patient relationship, since, many times, the professional comes to believe more in the request for complementary tests than in a well-done clinical examination. As already written by Lown[7]:

One reason for this situation is the introduction of increasingly sophisticated technologies. In comparison with the sharp images produced by ultrasound, magnetic resonance, computed tomography, endoscopy and angiography, the patient's report is insecure, confused, subjective and apparently irrelevant. In addition, obtaining a complete report takes a long time. According to some doctors, the technology has replaced the conversation with the patient.

And yet, according to the same author:

... the art of listening is the essence of the art of medicine practiced at the bedside. Listening carefully involves all the senses, not just the ears. The practice of the art of medicine requires not only the knowledge acquired about the disease, but also the appreciation of the intimate details of the patient's emotional life, which is generally assumed to be the psychiatrist's terrain. The need for complex involvement with the patient is never mentioned in the medical textbooks or mentioned in the training of professionals. To be successful in healing, the doctor needs to be trained above all else to listen. Just listening attentively has a therapeutic effect, as it provides knowledge of interesting stories. There are few books that expose the human condition more clearly than the patient that allows us to look deeply into his eyes.

On the other hand, over-specialization has led to the loss of the notion of the human being as a whole, starting to see him fragmented, as if his skin, or his bones, or joints, were not part of a single person. We know today that a good part of the diseases has systemic impairment and that each patient reacts in his own way to the illnesses. This lack of a holistic view is also a consequence of ignorance of the history of medicine.

According to Edgar Morin[8], "Hyperspecialization prevents both the perception of the global (which it fragments into portions) and of the essential (which it dissolves). It prevents even correctly treating particular problems, which can only be proposed and thought about in their context".

To believe, however, that higher education can be modified, without, at the same time, profound changes taking place in the models currently governing the training of health professionals, would be a demonstration of considerable naivety and lack of pragmatism. The approach to change must be systemic, ranging from curricula and teaching methods to student performance and competence assessment systems[9].

Aside from this, the evolution of genetic engineering, assisted reproduction, the artificial maintenance of certain vital functions and organ transplants, in addition to other scientific achievements, has led to the discussion of several issues of an ethical nature and of marked importance for the future of humanity.

For Heidegger[10], modern man finds himself in a situation of helplessness due to the break in tradition caused by the development of modern science and the dominance of technology in Western culture. Nihilism, which characterizes part of current civilization and which has contributed to the increase in drug use with its negative repercussions, such as the increase in violence in large cities[11], would be a consequence of the death of tradition.

Another way of approaching this question was how the anthropologist Claude Lévi-Straus said: "The moment that man knows no limit to his power, he begins his self-destruction". [12]

Polish philosopher Leszek Kolakowski also made an important contribution to this debate when he said: "To be completely free from any sense, to be totally free from tradition, is to be in a void and, therefore, to explode, pure and simple. The utopia of total autonomy and the hope of unlimited perfection are perhaps the most effective instruments of suicide that human culture has ever invented."[13]

There are several ways to present the history of health sciences. There are books of hundreds of pages, with numerous sequences of names and dates. There are still others who seek to share this account through the centuries. Another way was used by Bynum[14], in which medicine is divided into five types: at the bedside (or aimed at home care), theoretical (or linked to studies and at universities), hospital, social (or community-oriented) and laboratory (and linked more to the research area, using laboratory animals or even humans, as in the case of therapeutic trials).

Another way that could be more reasonable and interesting to make this description would be to try to detect its most remarkable moments.

According to Thomas Kuhn[15], scientific research can be divided into periods of relatively quiet development, interspersed with periods of major change, or of real revolutions in the field of science. During a given period, knowledge is governed by a generally accepted paradigm.

The paradigm, essentially a conceptual framework involving both theory and practice, allows the accommodation of new knowledge that will be acquired over time, until a new framework or paradigm no longer allows this accommodation to continue to be made.

This whole structure is put down after the emergence of a new conceptual framework. An example of how a revolution like this occurred in the field of biology was Darwin's evolutionary theory, which completely overthrew the theory that each species had been created independently, that is, that the characteristics of species were fixed.

Three moments in the history of the art of healing were fundamental, according to several authors, serving, as a consequence, as milestones of different periods of their development:

> • The first was the publication of Andreas Vesalius' anatomy book, *De humani corporis fabrica*, in 1543, when teaching the surgical bases of medicine changed from a speculative method based on the study of the anatomy of animals to a scientific and supported method in the dissection of human corpses.
> • The second important moment was the germ theory, developed by Louis Pasteur, in 1862, which annulled, definitively, the theory of spontaneous generation, accepted since antiquity.
> • The third milestone in this story was the discovery of

the helical structure of deoxyribonucleic acid (DNA) by James Dewey Watson and Francis Harry Crick, in 1953, and later, the genetic code. From that period onwards, the health sciences took a qualitative leap whose consequences, in the future, are impossible to evaluate today.

The last part of this work seeks to rescue some moments that were lost with time. It is interesting, because it reproduces true classics from the history of science, and how some diseases were treated until the beginning of the 20th century.

Some personalities are presented through their own reports, which contributes to enrich the period in which they developed their research and obtained their achievements.

A conclusion that can be drawn when reading this text is that mankind owes not only to doctors the great transformation that the art of healing has undergone, from the most remote times to the present day.

Lawyers, teachers, journalists, engineers, physicists, chemists, pharmacists, dentists, physiotherapists, nutritionists, veterinarians, nurses, biologists, psychologists and even professionals with no higher education, such as the Dutchman Leeuwenhoek, inventor of the microscope, made a considerable contribution to the development of this noble art.

In addition, countless anonymous people whose names will never be remembered, but who also made an important contribution to research and the evolution of health sciences, even through their simple daily work, are also worthy of respect and admiration.

I also dedicate this book to them. The primitive art of cure

Medicine can be defined as the art of dealing with the phenomenon of love, proper to the body. Plato, *The Banquet*

The beginning
─────────

When humanity, in its early days, lived in harmony with nature - and when it dominated the human spirit, and not the other way around - the healing processes were essentially empirical.

It was in this magical way that medicine developed. In its popular manifestation it remains, even today, in close relationship with the learning of the diverse forces of nature on the one hand and beliefs in magic on the other.

By observing the primitive peoples of today, we have a faithful portrait of the life forms of human beings in the most remote past.

Some claim that fear created religious feeling[16]. The fragility of man in the face of nature, diseases and the other difficulties of his miserable existence made him lacking the supernatural, as a form of protection in the midst of such an adverse scenario.

In its origin, the practice of magic is confused with that of religion, focusing on some individuals who came to be considered as having extraordinary powers.

On the day the first magician appeared, the first priest and the first doctor also appeared.

Consequently, it would be natural for those who practiced primitive medicine to be the same ones who, knowing the fragility of the human being and the virtues of plants and the poisons of animals, also started to attribute powers differentiated from the others. Those who, possessed of fantastic faculties, were said to be able to summon the spirits of the dead or to appease them.

The practice of their functions makes them mediators between man and the gods, which leads them to achieve the greatest divine attribute of all time, the power over life and death and the ability to cure diseases.

The growing knowledge allows them to become more and more powerful.

Thus, to keep their secrets and maintain their source of dominance, they constitute a caste - linked by special rites - and, frequently, by a complicated and secret initiation system.

Periodically, they perform ceremonies of sacrifices or bloody rites, for the recognition of the importance of blood as a source of life, since the first hunters believed that the animals' souls were in their blood, starting from there also the belief that by this means they could appropriate up the enemy's life force.

Or, still, they perform surgeries, such as skull trepanizations - performed since the Neolithic period -, or the mutilation and castration surgeries used today in primitive African tribes, which remove the clitoris of increasingly younger girls.

An atmosphere of mystery surrounds them. Colorful garments, sacred amulets, animal skins and other fetishes contribute to differentiate them from others.

But, behind all this apparent simplicity, there is a dose of wisdom. Whether as a result of accumulated experience, through suggestion or the use of plants - therapeutic activity recognized today - they are able to carry out their healing processes.

Finally, it can be said that medicine originated at the same time as civilization, not as a science, but as a belief that it was a gift given by the gods.

The Chinese art of healing

China has the oldest medical texts we know. The father of Chinese medicine, Fu-Hsi, lived about 2900 years ago, and invented the fundamental philosophy of yang and yin.

Then, about 200 years later, Shen-Nung appeared. His work, *Pen Tsao Kang Mu* (*Classification of Roots and Herbs*), deals mainly with the vegetable pharmacopoeia with a description of over a thousand drugs, some of which are still used today.

Another contribution of Chinese medicine is the use of iron (for anemia), arsenic (for intermittent fevers), mercury (in the treatment of some infections) and opium (for pain). Also from China, are the oldest records on infusions obtained with a plant (Ma Huang) used to treat asthma, which, today, is known to have ephedrine as an active component. The substance produces dilation of the bronchial tree, despite increasing the heart rate.

Another important plant for the Chinese was ginseng. They believed that there would be a substance that enhanced virility. From their roots, they made teas that should be drunk for eight consecutive days. They also recommended that the root should also be ingested in order to obtain a greater therapeutic effect.

Emperor Huang-Ti, who lived around 2600 BC, was the author of the book *Nei Ching* (*Doctrine of the Interior*). It is about the reconstitution of dialogues between the emperor and one of his ministers, Chi Po. The dialogues addressed the functions of the human body, its diseases and its cures.

It is interesting to note, in this work, the statement that the blood of the human body would be under the control of the heart and would be regulated by it; and that blood circulates continuously, which was only confirmed by William Harvey in the 17th century.

Another contribution of Chinese medicine was the belief that the body was formed by five elements, or by five types of processes, each represented by an archetype: earth, fire, water, wood and metal. Health would be due to the harmony between such elements. This conception came, later, to influence the Greek medicine of Antiquity, whose theory of humors (liquids or basic elements of the organism) originates from this formula created by the Chinese and also by the Indians.

The human body would be a miniature of the universe and would consist of the same materials as that universe. The disease should be seen more as a disharmony between man and his environment. Traditional Chinese medicine makes no difference between physical illness and mental illness, mental illness resulting from the loss of harmony between body and spirit.

The five elements would correspond not only to organs, but also to planets. Thus, the heart, liver, spleen, lungs and kidneys would be associated, respectively, with the elementary processes symbolized by fire, wood, earth, metal and water, as well as with the planets Mars, Jupiter, Saturn, Venus and Mercury.

Like other peoples of antiquity, the Chinese were weak in anatomy, due to the prohibition on dissecting corpses. They believed that if the body was not kept intact, the deceased could not be received in the realm of the dead.

Chinese medicine also seeks a balance between the yin (feminine, passive, negative principle, corresponding to the moon, the earth, the darkness, the delicacy, the wet, the cold and the right side) and the yang (masculine, active, positive, corresponding to the sun, the sky, the light, the power, the dry, the hot and the left side). There is also yin therapy, such as treatments with medicinal plants, and yang therapy, such as acupuncture and moxibustion.

According to Taoist legend, the god who formed the universe was successful after dividing chaos into its two opposite elements, yang and yin.

Through the search for balance between the two opposing principles, health was maintained and the disease was cured. In a way, yang and yin could represent the antagonism between the two components of the autonomic nervous system, the sympathetic and the parasympathetic. This is the part of the nervous system that is independent of our will and that is responsible for controlling our internal organs.

The dialectical interaction of opposites is one of the most important elements for understanding the nature of the creation and development of civilizations. Not only did the Chinese realize the importance of this phenomenon, but after them, also the Indians and then the Greeks, in the form of love and hate, until we arrived at Hegel with his theory of thesis and antithesis.

Chinese doctors focused on examining their patients' pulse

and tongue inspection to make their diagnoses, prognosis and treatments. The pulse examination value would be equivalent to that of a musical string instrument. In him, they believed, they could recognize harmonies and disharmonies. The examination of the pulse was done in eleven different parts of the body.

Another interesting contribution of Chinese medicine was a primitive technique of trying to immunize against smallpox, which consisted of making young people inhale the scabs of sick lesions, in the hope that in this way they would develop some type of resistance against smallpox. The boys aspirated the lesions with the left nostril and the girls with the right nostril, respecting the principles of yang and yin.

Two other important contributions of Chinese medicine, still used today, are the technique of acupuncture and moxibustion. The technique of acupuncture, with long needles, is based on the idea that the body is full of tubes similar to channels, a natural idea for the Chinese, whose agriculture was based on irrigation by channels.

Acupuncture uses iron, silver or gold needles, of variable dimensions, which are inserted into the skin, in some of the 360 points distributed in twelve meridians - or nerve paths - that travel through the body and transmit vital energy, or *chi* .

An internal component (viscera, bone, joint) corresponds to each territory of the skin, starting from there the correspondence between the meridians and the search for the balance that acunputura seeks to restore, since for the Chinese everything that exists in the universe is associated.

The ear has an energetic structure linked directly to the organs, according to acupuncturists. There are 200 auricular points. Placed in these ear points, the needles would have a great therapeutic effect.

In the end, acupuncture seeks to restore the balance between the two opposing principles of life, allowing one or the other to overflow, and reactivating blocked connections. Needle bites also release analgesic substances, endorphins, which increase pain tolerance.

Moxibustion uses the same meridians as acupuncture, but instead of needles heat is applied through a paper straw, where the dried herb of sagebrush is burned.

Recently recognized as a medical specialty, acupuncture has been used to treat everything from spinal problems to anxiety. The analgesia thus obtained is currently considered a more adequate alternative than that of anesthesia in Western medicine for elderly patients, or those with some serious underlying disease, and who need to undergo some type of surgery.

In the 20th century, a new form of treatment was developed in Japan, *shiatsu,* which combines manual stimulation with pressure on acupuncture points and meditation to relax the body and treat chronic pain.

The Chinese were the introductors of forensic medicine, in the year 1247 of the Christian era, when Judge Sung Tzu presented a treaty involving medicine and law entitled *Hsi Yüan Lu* (Instructions to Magistrates responsible for investigating deaths suspected of being crimes). The book contained information for the accurate verification of the signs present in the different causes of unnatural death, such as drowning, poisoning, strangulation, injuries by sharp objects or by bruises. It also presented methods to understand the differences between suicides and homicides, in addition to containing instructions on artificial respiration and the use of antidotes against some poisons.

The Mesopotamian art of healing

The first medical text of Western civilization appeared in the third Ur dynasty, from 2,158 to 2008 BD. In Mesopotamia, where today is Iraq. It is a clay tablet from the Sumerians, where it was recommended, for the treatment of wounds, the association of wine, prunes, juniper (plant from which gin is extracted) and a lot of beer. This mixture was then held close to the body, like a plaster.

Herodotus[17], the great historian of Antiquity, thus describes the beginning of medical practice among the Mesopotamians: "They brought their patients to the market place, because they had no doctors; then those who passed by the sick person, talked to him about his illness to find out if they themselves would not have been afflicted by the same evil as that person, or if they would have seen others like that. Then, the passerby checked with him and recommended that he could succeed with the same treatment with which he would have escaped the disease, or also if they had met others who would have been cured; and they were not allowed to pass by a sick person in silence, without inquiring about the nature of their indisposition".

It was in Babylon, during the reign of Hammurabi (1948 to 1905 BC), that the first civil and criminal liability code of the medical profession emerged. Article 215 of the Code provided:

- If the doctor successfully performs a major operation or heals a free man's sick eye, he should receive ten silver coins.

- If you are a slave, you should receive two silver coins.

- If the patient is a free citizen and the doctor causes him to lose his life or an eye on the operation, the doctor should have his hands cut off.

- If the misfortune occurs with a slave, the doctor must replace it with another slave.

In the great library of Nineveh, King Assurbanipal, of Assyria (669 to 626 BC), collected thousands of clay tablets, 800 of which dealt with health issues. Reading these texts, it is evident that, at the time, demons were considered an important cause of diseases.

For their treatments the Mesopotamians used fruits, leaves, flowers, bark and roots of various plants. They also used minerals such as copper and iron, as well as a lot of filth, in the belief that, with this, they displeased the demons and made them leave the sick body. They used various types of preparations: pills, powders, enemas.

The Babylonians reached a high degree of cultural development: they knew the periodicity of eclipses; they knew the position of the planets in relation to the sun; watched the passage of meteors; they had knowledge of mathematics, architecture and sculpture.

Babylonian medicine was heavily influenced by astrology. They believed that everything depended on metaphysical forces related to the stars. Just as the stars influenced the forces of nature, such as the movement of the tides that depends on the changes of the Moon, the moods of the human body should also be influenced by the stars.

It is possible that they affected other later civilizations with their beliefs, especially with this association between medicine, astronomy and astrology.

The Egyptian art of healing

Imhotep, the god of medicine of the Egyptians, is well before Asclepius, god of medicine of the Greeks. Some go so far as to say that he really did exist, having been born in about 2,700 BC and that he was probably a priest and an expert in the art of healing. According to Durant[18], Imhotep would have been appointed by Pharaoh Zoser as its main minister, in 2680 a. Ç.

Several temples and monuments were built in honor of this great curator, like a stone structure near the city of Memphis, where there is a step pyramid in Sakkara, considered the mother of all pyramids. The name Imhotep means "who comes in peace".

Medicine in ancient Egypt, as well as in Mesopotamia, was under the responsibility of the priests and was taught in schools located next to the temples of Imhotep. The main ones were in the cities of On, Memphis, Lais and Theben.

What is known about Egyptian medicine is found in the papyri dating from 2200 to 1800 BC, written in the 12th dynasty. Those found in the Egyptian locality of Kahun deal only with women's illnesses. Other papyri from 1700 to 1500 BC, written in the early 18th dynasty, were much better preserved.

The latter are called Ebers papiros, because they were acquired by Prof. Georg Ebers[19], who was born in 1837 in Germany, has -If Egyptologist in Jena in 1865 , and professor in Leipzig in 1870.

In 1873, he bought a massive roll of papyrus, twenty meters long, from an American resident in Egypt, Edwin Smith, an antique dealer.

The scroll would have been found next to a mummy and Thebes in 1862 and should have been written around 1550 BC

With content written on both sides, present a mixture of magic formulas, recipes for the preparation of medicines, clinical observations and treatments for injuries caused by trauma.

Among the diseases described in papyrus, hematuria (presence of blood in the urine) is frequent. Later, it can be seen that these were cases of bladder schistosomiasis (bilharzia), a disease caused by *Shistosoma haematobium*, a parasitosis still common in Egypt today.

The rains were relatively rare, but not the floods caused by the Nile. Each year, the river surpassed its banks, covering the land on either side of its bed for more than two kilometers. To irrigate as much land as possible, in a region where drought was common, farmers created a complex system of channels to dam the waters of the Nile.

Periodically, there was an enormous amount of stagnant water in these channels, an ideal breeding ground not only for the development of parasites such as schistosomiasis but also for vectors such as mosquitoes, thus allowing malaria to be another very common communicable disease among the Egyptians, as evidenced by study conducted at the Anthropological Museum in Turin, Italy.

Using molecular biology techniques, researchers were able to detect a specific protein from *Plasmodium falciparum* (PfHRP2) in 21 out of 50 mummies tested and which showed signs of anemia, such as splenomegaly and porotic cranial hyperostosis.

Tuberculosis was also a frequent disease, although the papyri did not mention it. Studies of the bones of mummies allowed the detection of several cases of bone tuberculosis, causing lesions of the vertebral bodies, resulting in kyphosis and buckling of the spine, a lesion known as Pott's disease.

Magic was a prominent part of the Egyptian social and religious life. It affected not only the relations of men with their neighbors, but also with the dead and the gods. According to them, magic was a means of achieving their needs and desires.

The disease was seen as a consequence of the possession of a demon, or of a poison that the evil being would have introjected into the victim's body. Once installed, the demon would make the person sick and what the doctor should try to do, first, was to expel the invader.

In medical papyri, interspersed with drug prescriptions, it is possible to observe the citation of magic words, which would serve to make medicines more effective.

Some of these "drugs", or procedures, would be mere absurd, were it not for their own logical explanation. This is the case of coprotherapy, the excrement intake prescribed as a way to expel the evil spirit that inhabited the patient's body.

While the Babylonians believed the liver to be the seat of life and the center of blood circulation, the Egyptians considered breathing to be the most important vital function and admitted the image of mobile air, pneuma, as its essential principle.

The well-known cult of the dead, with advanced embalming techniques, was due to the belief in the existence of life after death, and this required the conservation of the dead body in the best possible way.

The embalming practice consisted of the following: the brain was first removed with a hook through the nostrils; then an opening was made in the abdomen, with a sharp knife, to remove all the viscera from the cavity, which was then filled with myrrh, cassia leaves and other resins mixed with the incense, closing the corpse, then through sewing.

Then the body was immersed in natural soda for seventy days. Then it was washed, wrapped in bandages made of fine linen fabric , with a layer of gum. Finally, the body was handed over to the family, who placed it in a wooden coffin, in human form, to later be placed in the burial chamber.

After they died, the pharaohs were buried with everyone around them, so that they could continue to serve them in the hereafter. Together with their tombs, they stored food and great treasures in the belief that they would continue to enjoy, after reincarnation, everything they had become accustomed to.

Egyptian medicine combined empirical rationalism with mysticism. The Egyptians had a high degree of progress in the field of hygiene. Details were made for the burial of the dead and strict rules existed to guide the cleaning of the rooms, the preparation of meals and even for sexual relations. The entire life of the Egyptians was regulated by precise laws, covered in the form of religious elements. In Egyptian medicine, religious regulations and hygienic recommendations are often confused.

The priests could only wear white clothes, and avoided some

types of food such as pork. The water could only be drunk if it was boiled or filtered. Egyptian law severely punished artificial abortion and child abandonment. It also prohibited the practice of sexual intercourse during menstruation and considered masturbation to be a shameful addiction.

The Egyptians were the initiators of urotherapy, that is, the therapeutic use of urine, according to papyrus of the 15th century BC, where a formula for burns consisting of pumpkin seeds, salt and urine is prescribed. Today we know that urine contains a series of substances with biological activity, such as urea (the main form of nitrogen elimination by the body), urokinase (an enzyme capable of dissolving clots), antibodies, sex hormones and other molecules.

According to Heródoto, there was a great specialization among the doctors of ancient Egypt, with doctors for the treatment of women's diseases, eye diseases, diseases caused by trauma and specialists in "unknown diseases", which would be diseases whose causes were not known and for which the magical formulations would be indicated.

Circumcision was widely used and generally performed when boys reached the age of 14.

As a wound dressing, an association of myrrh and honey was used, bandaged with linen, for a period of four days. Honey has antimicrobial activity, because there is an enzyme inside that, acting on glucose and oxygen, produces hydrogen peroxide, with a potent action on various types of bacteria and fungi. The fact that honey is a substance capable of carrying water and leading microbial cells to desiccation (dehydrating the internal environment) also contributes to increasing its effectiveness.

The Egyptians also used onions, garlic and radishes, which are now recognized to have some infection-fighting properties.

For birth control, they used various methods, such as the use of a pessary, or circular artifact similar to the current diaphragm, which obstructs the cervix, and also the ingestion of resins such as myrrh and sap, or of plants such as mugwort and rue.

They also made strange remedies from pigs' crystals, lizard blood, lion's brains and women's milk. They also used purgatives, diuretics, emetics, sweat and expectorants, since they were also adept at humoral theory.

There is a quote, in one of the more recent papyri, that says: "Heal him with the knife and then burn him with the fire that he will no longer bleed." This recommendation was later followed by the Greeks, who recommended the use of cautery in surgeries.

The Hebrew Art of Healing

The medicine of the Hebrews can be known through the Bible (Old Testament) and the Talmud, sacred book, where the tradition of religion is registered until today followed by the rabbis.

In the secular sense, the great contribution of Hebrew medicine concerns hygiene and public health.

On the other hand, here the disease is still considered as a result of divine wrath, and the cessation of suffering can only be obtained through prayers, fasting and observance of moral laws.

Consequently, there is a tendency to concentrate all healing capacity in the hands of the priests, who are the intermediaries of the will of one God. They also see illnesses as a purifying process for the soul and body.

The study of medical knowledge through the Bible is disappointing, according to Guthrie[20] : "In the Old Testament there is a small place for the doctor, if there was such a place, because there God is responsible for the healings".

This people, which, for the first time in history, ensures equal rights for all individuals, provided they obey their strict moral laws and religious foundations, also for the first time establishes the concept of health legislation, where the collective interest predominates over the individual. In times of frequent and terrible epidemics, this new concept was very important for the preservation of the Jewish people.

Among the main recommendations of Judaism regarding health are hygienic practices (to get in touch with God it was always necessary to be clean), the practice of circumcision (which brings less possibility of contracting venereal diseases and cancer of the penis), and the prohibition eating pork (due to the risk, known today, of teniasis and cysticercosis). He also created a weekly day of rest, the Sabbath.

Some examples of recommended practices in the Old Testament:

Anyone who wanted to defecate had to leave the camp, taking a small shovel to bury their feces.

Everyone should wash before and after meals, and after sexual contact. Any type of abnormal secretion from Organs sexual organs made the carrier "impure", so that he was required to leave the camp.

Anyone who touched a person, who was believed to have died of an infectious disease, was required to be isolated for seven days. After this period, it should be purified with a solution of potash, hyssop and cedar.

The warriors who returned to the camp, after having maintained contact with other peoples or tribes, needed to be isolated for eight days.

Rigid measures like these allowed the Hebrews to survive the difficult and long crossing of the desert. Started from the year 1500 BC[21], and guided by Moses, the journey took forty years to complete. To a large extent, the medicine of the Hebrews was influenced by the Egyptians and Mesopotamians.

The Indian art of healing

The history of Indian medicine is divided into three periods:

An older period, which goes from 1500 to 800 BC, called the Vedic period because the information is derived mainly from the Vedas (word meaning knowledge), the four sacred Sanskrit books of the Indians: Rig-Veda, Sama-Veda, Yajur-Veda, and Atarva-Veda. The Vedas are ancient hymns, philosophical-religious poems, prayers and teachings from the Aryan peoples, who invaded the Indus valley around 1500 BC

A later period, or Brahmanic, that goes from 800 to 600 BC, and the Brahminism received a strong influence from the religion of the Aryan peoples who conquered India. They had a caste system that was perpetuated in Brahminism, in addition to transforming the forces of nature into human-looking gods. Its main deities were Indra (god of time and war), Varuna (god of water), Agni (god of fire) and Soma (god of hallucinogenic plants).

It is a period called Buddhist, which goes from 600 BC to 600 AD, after which large parts of India were subjected to Islam, and Arab medicine, as a result, came to exert great influence in the country.

The Brahmanic period has this designation because it is based on the culture dominated by the caste of the priests of this religion, as well as the Buddhist period, dominated by its monks.

The first, or Vedic, period corresponds to that of the most primitive medicine.

The Brahmanic period presents a more rational basis, and Hindu medicine reached its peak in the Buddhist period, where medical education started to have a more elaborate theoretical and practical training, similar to the Greek medicine of Antiquity.

Traditional Indian medicine, also known as Ayurve da, considers that there are fluids in the body, called *doshas*. The first, *vata*, is characterized by being dry, cold and light. The second, *pitta,* hot, bitter and pungent. The third, *kapha,* cold, heavy and sweet. They are fundamental for the correct functioning of the body when there is an excess or lack of one or more of them, or when they are taught in inadequate topography, diseases occur.

The three classic books of Indian medicine are the bocks of Charaka (beginning of the Christian era), Susruta (around 500 AD) and Vagbhata (around 600 AD).

Charaka cataloged more than 500 remedies, classifying them into five groups, according to the nature of his action: tonics, sedatives, laxatives, purgatives, emetics and aphrodisiacs.

Susruta is considered the father of Indian surgery. Identified 1.120 diseases, classifying them into seven groups. He described eight types of surgical interventions: incision, puncture, drilling, scarification, extraction, suture, excision, and drainage.

Vagbhata, who was born in Sindh, today Pakistan's province, wrote a tract known as *Astanga Hrdaya*, in three volumes, having received his Ayurvedic medicine teachings from his father and a Buddhist monk, called Avalokita.

His work is divided into the following sections: Internal Medicine, Pediatrics, Gynecology, Psychiatry, Toxicology, Basic Surgery, Rejuvenation Therapy and Geriatrics.

In addition to being a clearer summary of the texts by Charaka and Susruta, his work also includes new information that did not exist in previous texts, such as longevity, personal hygiene, causes of diseases, influences of seasons and time on the human organism, pregnancy and possible complications during childbirth, as well as various indications on how to establish a prognosis and how to treat certain diseases.

In Indian medicine, the disease was also considered as a divine punishment, but the belief in reincarnation, originating from Buddhism, brought something new to this association.

According to tradition, in the 6th century BC, Siddartha Gautama, a young prince who would later be known as Buddha, "the enlightened one", left his parents' house, at the age of 29, in search of a life of poverty and asceticism. After a series of failed experiences, at the foot of a fig tree, he finally realized his great revelation, which consisted of discovering the cause of pain in the world and the path to be followed for his liberation: only the perfect state of happiness would be reached through suppression of all forms of desire and satisfaction of bodily desires, in addition to the annihilation of human personality[22].

Siddartha recommended "that man overcome anger by goodness and evil by good. May hatred never end in hatred; may hatred end in love ". Despite all this capacity for bestowal and detachment, he never claimed that a god spoke through him. Its five moral rules recommended: do not kill any living thing; not taking what is not offered; do not lie; do not drink intoxicating drinks; and not be impure.

According to Buddha, the human being would be continually being reborn, until his "karma" - that is, the set of actions in the life of each one that determined his destiny - would lead him to Nirvana, eternal peace, or the merger with the universe, the which represents nothing more than the eternal cycle of creation, development and destruction, followed after new creation and so indefinitely, something similar to the current big bang theory of creating the universe.

Nirvana would not represent paradise after death, but the liberation of the soul from all selfishness, or from the absurdity of individualism that generates the evils of the world. According to Buddha, when we learn to love all beings, and not only our isolated selves, we find Nirvana or altruistic peace.

For Siddartha, nothingness would be the beginning of all things, everything would arise out of nothing and return there.

The Hindu religious attitude towards animals, closely linked to the "karma" theory, probably explains why human and veterinary medicine were not separate.

Yoga, derived from Ayurvedic medicine, is a deistic philosophy. Through the practice of meditation and exercises, it aims to suppress all activity of the body and mind, in order to allow to release the spirit of the body. Yoga practitioners must seek the way to overcome all kinds of suffering and, with the rupture of the oppressive connection of each one to the physical world, achieve a spiritual state of enlightenment and liberation of the body.

The difficulty in studying Indian medicine lies in being able to separate fact from fiction in its primitive documents.

In the Rig-Veda, about 1500 years BC, it is described that the treatment of diseases at that time consisted mainly of magic and sorcery. The following work, called Atarva-Veda, contains much more information. Various diseases have been described, such as malaria, tuberculosis and smallpox. There are also descriptions of 760 medicinal plants.

They were adepts of the humoral theory, being the body constituted by four elements: air, mucus, bile and blood. The disease was seen as a consequence of the alteration of the balance between the constituent elements of the body. It could also develop due to external causes, such as accidents and possessions by demons, curses and witchcraft.

Against illnesses caused by sins (done in this or another past life) they prescribed penances, prayers and the payment of promises as the only forms of therapy.

The Indian doctor was the first to describe diabetes and tasted the urine of all patients. They were very advanced in diagnostic techniques. The physical examination included examination of the wrist, ear, palpation and auscultation.

They introduced cataract surgery and lithotomy surgery to remove bladder stones.

Another contribution of Indian medicine was in the development of plastic surgery. Rhinoplasty was widely performed, since under criminal law, the punishment of various crimes was punished by amputating the ear and nose. This was common in crimes of adultery, with only women being punished in this way. The leaf of a tree was used to serve as a template to cut a piece of skin from the forehead or forearm, which was then sutured at the amputation site.

Women were only accepted as midwives, which was no different from other societies. They only started to be admitted as doctors from the 14th century, in Europe.

The Greek art of healing

The importance of Hellenic culture in Western civilization is unquestionable. In philosophy, politics, theater, architecture, mathematics, just to name a few examples, the Greeks exercised and still exercise a strong influence on our civilization today. There is nothing more natural than in medicine, this ascendancy has been significant.

Greek culture originated from the Minoan civilization, from the island of Crete. Protected from invaders by the Mediterranean, the Greeks were skilled navigators, who extended their influence mainly across the Aegean. They constituted a peaceful society and turned to commercial activity.

With their reflexive way of seeing the world, the

Greeks created philosophy, on the other hand, rejecting the religious prevalence of myth, in addition to admitting the diversity of rational interpretations of each phenomenon.

Thus, Greek civilization was essentially secular and rationalist. He exalted free thinking and placed knowledge above faith. He was almost completely indifferent to what would happen to them after death. The Greeks believed that when they died, they went to the dark kingdom of Hades, located under the earth, but that no one was punished or rewarded for what he had done in life.

With the book *Elements,* Euclides, around 300 BC. C., gave considerable contribution to Mathematics. Divided into 13 parts called "Books", the text deals especially with flat geometry. Euclides' work also shows how to think in a logical way on any subject, that is, how to build, step by step, a complex theory, which came to considerably influence the thinking of several philosophers and scientists, such as Descartes, Spinoza, Gottfried Leibniz and Isaac Newton[23].

Thales de Mileto (625 to 548 BC), surprisingly, predicted the sun's eclipse of 585 BC, based on his astronomical studies. This gave him great credibility, and through his teachings he managed to destroy myths and superstitions that involved diseases. In those days, the prophecies and prognosis of diseases were given by the oracles, or by examining the liver of sacrificed animals. Thales is also attributed with the statement that the sum of the angles of a triangle is equal to two right angles and that the sides of similar triangles are proportional. Thales also made another important contribution in attributing water to the material origin of all things.

In addition to Thales, the initial scientific basis for Greek medicine was given by Pythagoras[24] (580 to 497 BC), which also contributed to removing the supernatural mantle that existed until then from the disease. This thinker, still known today by the theorem that bears his name, established that the principles of harmony and proportion governed the universe, reflecting the macrocosm. The same should also happen with our body, or microcosm. Pythagoras is also credited with the first mention of the spherical shape of the Earth.

Aristotle, another important name in the early days of medicine, was the son of a doctor, and wrote three great works of biology: the *history of animals*, *parts of animals* and *generation of animals*.

He also made an important contribution to the nature of life itself. For him, the difference between living and non-living matter did not depend on its material constitution, but on the presence or absence of something he called the psyche, which could be translated by soul or conscience. Aristotle was one of the greatest sages of antiquity, and in the field of medicine he is also considered the founder of comparative anatomy for his studies on the anatomy of vertebrates and invertebrates[25].

Hippocrates was the best known Greek physician and the one who had the most prestige accumulated throughout history. There are testimonies about his real existence given by Plato and Aristotle, and he considered Hippocrates the most perfect type of doctor he met.

Born on the island of Kos (450 to 370 BC), he said that anyone who wanted to dedicate himself to medicine should have a vocation and a great capacity for dedication to work and study. Following the school of Pythagoras, he broke with magic and mysticism and gave medicine the first foundations of a rational science / art. Suggestion, belief and mystery are unworthy of the standard of conduct of doctors, he taught.

It started to give primary importance to the contact with the patient, being attributed to him the form, still used today, of how to make a consultation: consciously interrogate, listen, observe, make a physical exam, establish a diagnosis, make a prognosis and define the treatment.

His doctrine could be summed up with a phrase that he always repeated to his students: "each disease has a natural cause and without natural causes nothing happens". His classes were given in the shade of a plane tree, an ancient tree that still exists today on the island of Kos.

In a period when doctors often traveled from place to place, establishing an adequate prognosis was the best thing to do, since the cures happened more by nature's response than by the treatments used. This was one of the reasons for the fame of Hippocrates and other contemporaries of Greek medicine.

The Greeks of the 5th century BC believed that the universe was formed by four elements: water, earth, fire and air[26]. Each of these elements corresponded to intrinsic qualities: humidity and cold for water, dryness and cold for earth, heat and dryness for fire and heat and humidity for air.

Hippocrates developed a theory, influenced by the other cultures that preceded that of the Greeks, according to which the organism consists of four types of moods: blood, mucus, yellow bile and black bile. The blood was characterized by being warm and dry. The cold, moist mucus. Hot and wet yellow bile, and cold, dry black bile. The blood would originate in the heart, mucus in the brain, yellow bile in the liver and black bile in the spleen.

In order to be healthy, there was a need to balance these moods. The excess or lack of any of them would produce the disease. This would also have to do with the treatment of illnesses.

If one of the moods, such as blood, was in a larger volume than necessary, bleeding should be performed and balance and, consequently, health would be restored.

This was the basis for the use of medicines of the time: bleeding, purging and vomiting, enemas, herbs, laxatives and hot baths, in order to induce bleeding, vomiting, diarrhea and sweating.

They assumed that eliminating excess humor would restore lost health. There was also a recommendation to use diets and exercise.

It was also Hippocrates who gave the ethical foundations of the profession. In the famous oath that medical students still repeat today - and in which the Greek gods are mentioned, Apollo, physician of the gods and father of Asclepius (Esculapius in Latin), god of medicine, who in turn was the father of Hygia, goddess of health, and Panacea, goddess of healing -, formulates some of the still respected precepts of the medical code of ethics, such as not causing harm to patients, not having sexual relations with the patient and their family members, not practicing euthanasia, not practicing abortion, keep secret what you hear from your customers, respect your masters and your disciples, and maintain behavior worthy of your professional activity.

Greek medical schools developed next to the Asclepius temples, where there was an abundance of sick people, because the sick went there after their cures.

The journey of the sick to the temples, in fact, was not to be treated as it is known today.

They went to sleep in the temple to dream of Asclepius himself, who during the dream would reveal to them what to do to treat their illnesses.

When the sick could not, by themselves, understand the meaning of dreams, the temple priests interpreted them and told them what should be done. In fact, the medicine capable of performing the cures was the faith brought by each one who came to seek help. It is also interesting to note the importance they attached to the meaning of dreams, which long after came to be emphasized with the foundation of psychoanalysis, by Freud.

The most famous medical schools in ancient Greece were those of Rhodas, Crotona, Kos and Cnido.

Every aspirant in the medical profession had to look for his own improvement, which he acquired in the form of private education (with other more experienced doctors) or attending traditional medical schools. No proof of sufficiency was required before the profession could be started. This resulted in many charlatans, which hindered the practice of doctors with adequate training.

It is believed that not everything that is attributed to Hippocrates was actually written by him, but by other doctors who lived in similar periods, such as Chrysippus, Eurypus and Praxagoras. Some of his well-known aphorisms, however, remain part of his work today, such as the following:

"Life is so short, and art is so great to be learned, the occasion fleeting, the experience misleading, and the judgment difficult."[27]

"Diseases that medicine does not cure, the knife cures; those that the knife does not heal, fire can heal; but those that are not even healed by fire must be incurable."

"People who, when coughing, expel foamy blood,

this blood comes from the lung".

"Unexpected fatigue indicates disease".

"When a convalescent eats well and doesn't get fat, it's an unfavorable sign."

"In all illnesses, maintaining lucid intelligence and a taste for food is a good sign; the opposite is bad ".

"Physics appears mainly between the ages of 18 and 35".

"In jaundice it is a bad sign that the liver will harden."

"It is easier to repair forces with liquid foods than with solids."

"Those who are fat are more exposed to sudden death than those who are thin."

"It is the forces of nature that cure diseases".

The works of Hippocrates, together with those of other ancient Greek doctors, were brought together in the great library of Alexandria, by Ptolemy, one of the generals of Alexander the Great, Macedonian king and who had Aristotle as his preceptor, his education being worthy of man. who took it over. According to Hegel[28] Alexander favored the sciences and was, alongside Pericles, praised as the most generous protector of the arts of antiquity.

This information, contained in the so-called Hippocratic Collection, was estimated at a total of 131 works, dealing with the most diverse subjects, such as anatomy (an area in which the Greeks were disabled, since the dissection of corpses and their knowledge was forbidden based on in the study of animals), physiology, pathology, therapy, diagnosis, prognosis, surgery and obstetrics, among others.

Some books that are part of the Collection:

About ancient medicine - addresses the art of medicine from dietary practices and observations.

Epidemic diseases - mainly addresses diseases found on the island of Thasos.

On prognosis - reveals Hippocrates' deep knowledge of disease symptoms.

About the airs, waters and places - alerts the doctor what diseases you should know when entering a city, with certain climatic conditions. It is a classic of medical geography. It mentions, for the first time, the importance of environmental factors in the emergence of diseases.

The law and the doctor - addresses the professional attitude of the doctor and his ethical obligations.

The Alexandria School

The city of Alexandria has become the most important cultural center in antiquity.

In century III BD King Ptolemy II founded the famous library which, at its peak, had more than 500 thousand volumes or papyri. The *Museum* , or temple of the Muses as it was called, was much more than a simple library, being a true scientific and cultural center, for teaching and research, and also with an amphitheater, zoo, temple and observatory.

The library was first burned by the Romans in 47 and then in 390, by the bishop Teófilo, until finally being destroyed when the Arabs conquered Egypt in 642.

In medicine, in this important metropolis, Asclepíades, Heróphilo and Erasistrato emerged.

The school of Alexandria had as one of the main causes of its development the practice of dissecting the human body between the end of the third century BC until the beginning of the second century AD. This allowed a great development of anatomy and, consequently, of surgery.

Asclepíades said that the body was made of atoms, or elementary corpuscles imperceptible to the senses and that they continuously moved through the pores and channels of our body. He disagreed with Hippocrates' theory of moods. He considered that much more than medication, what should be done was to have healthy lifestyle habits. He was the first Greek doctor to be successful in Rome, having found in that society, idle and opulent, fertile ground for his preaching. He recommended diets, physical exercises, walks, baths and massages.

Heróphilo, of Chalcedon, was considered the greatest anatomist of Antiquity. He left a detailed description of the brain, the discovery of the meaning of the pulse and its use in the diagnosis of diseases, the distinction between tendons and nerves, and the relationship between them and the brain. Unlike Aristotle, who considered the heart to be the seat of intelligence and emotions (which continued to be true in literature for a long time), Heróphilo realized that the noblest functions of our body should be credited to the brain. He also believed in the theory of the moods of the oldest Greeks.

Erasistratus disagreed with this theory and believed that the activity of atoms came from the inspired air (pneuma, which meant the soul and the breath of life), which was distributed throughout the body through the arteries.

It was his information that the heart was the source of arteries and veins. Erasistratus, who left an important contribution in the field of anatomy, was accused of the practice of dissection in living criminals, vivisection.

It is known today that both Heróphilo and Erasístrato performed public dissection of human corpses.

The vivisection complaint made to Erasistratus and Heróphilo is due to Celso and Tertuliano (155 to 222 AD) and also to Saint Augustine (354 to 430 AD). Galeno, who was later to Heróphilo and Erasístrato, in none of his works corroborated these denunciations. Being so critical, and so contrary to Erasistratus's views, it is likely that these statements were false and actually portrayed a reaction to the practice of dissection in human corpses, which was condemned by the Church for many centuries.

The Roman art of healing

The most important of the Roman doctors was Aulus Cornelius Celsus, or Celso. He was the first to write his work in Latin, instead of Greek, as was the norm for scientific texts of the time. He wrote in perfect Latin, being extremely organized. There are doubts about his profession, since he wrote comprehensive works of knowledge of agriculture and military theory, and even of philosophy and law. The one dealing with medicine, *De res medica,* published in 30 AD, was the only one to survive, having been reprinted in the Middle Ages. It was Celso who, for the first time, defined the four signs of inflammation: pain, heat, redness and tumor. He also described several types of orthopedic treatments, such as reducing fractures and dislocations.

Caius Plinius Secundus, or Plínio the Elder (23 to 79 AD), also wrote a gigantic work, in 37 volumes, *Historia Natural*, dealing with subjects as varied as history, physics, chemistry, geography and medicine. It was, in fact, a compilation, which is supposed to be based on the writings of almost 500 different authors on various topics, which are still in use today.

Plínio was actually a journalist of his time. His legacy was a kind of popular encyclopedia, where everyone could appeal directly and always find some important information, stories or even advice. His books describe the customs, beliefs, superstitions and ideas of the time in which he lived.

Knowing that Vesuvius was erupting, he went to the city of Pompeii to check out the event for himself, as a good reporter he was. Even though he was warned of the danger he was in, he refused to leave the place.

On the third day he was there, after dinner he went to bed to rest for a while. Soon after, torrents of glowing lava fell on the city. His body was found intact three days later.

Apparently, he died intoxicated by the poisonous gases emitted by the volcano, during the eruption that destroyed Pompeii.

Pedanius Dioscórides (41 to 68 AD) was a doctor of Nero's armies, and had the opportunity to meet hundreds of plants during his travels with the military. He cataloged the plants according to the diseases they cured.

He elaborated a kind of pharmacopoeia, with the list of substances and remedies that medicine used to treat diseases. His book, *Hylikà* or *Materia Medica*, contained descriptions of 600 plants, presented beautiful drawings and was translated into several languages, having been used as a reference text for more than fifteen hundred years.

It consisted of five books: the first addressed aromatic substances, oil, ointments, trees and their juices, resins and fruits; the second dealt with animals, medicines of animal origin, vegetables and cereals; the third commented on herbs, roots and their juices, as well as seeds; the fourth book was about other herbs, roots and fungi; the fifth referred to wines and mineral remedies.

Dioscórides' work presents 500 remedies of vegetable origin, 35 of animal origin and 90 of mineral origin. He always followed the same principle regarding the presentation of medicines: characters of each substance, synonym, forgeries, evidence, actions and medical use.

Despite not having developed much the theory and practice of medicine, the Romans remained in history for their contributions in the field of public health.

They created a complex system of transporting and using water at a distance, which included reservoirs on hills, and which was served by aqueducts that transported the liquid to cisterns and from there to swimming pools or basins, where the sediment was deposited. This resulted in an improvement in the quality of water consumed in street fountains and in public bathhouses, which contributed to raising the population's level of personal hygiene. Some spas had accommodation, covered in marble, for up to three thousand people.

Between the 1st and 2nd centuries AD, that is, at its peak, Rome had a population of one million inhabitants. In order to take care of this urban agglomeration, ten large aqueducts supplied the Roman population with 40 million gallons of drinking water daily.

There was also a great concern about the fate of the waste. To solve the problem, a system for capturing rainwater and sewage through pipes under the streets was developed. These drained the water into a pipeline network of increasing caliber, until it ended in the maximum sewer, on the Tiber River.

In the 2nd century AD, a public health service was created to serve poor citizens who could not afford to pay doctors. In cities considered small, the State paid five doctors to serve the public. On average, seven, and for large companies, up to ten doctors were hired for this function.

Long before the discovery of microbes, the Romans were concerned with wet and swampy places. They tried to land these places, or to mix salt water with the pond, to inhibit the growth of mosquitoes, since they had noticed a strong association between swampy areas and diseases. Today, we know that mosquitoes transmit various diseases such as malaria, dengue and yellow fever.

With Rome, doctors constituted a class protected by the State, began to enjoy the esteem of the citizens, and came to occupy positions of the greatest political relevance. Even foreign doctors acquired rights similar to those of the Romans, were elevated to the top of the social scale and actively participated in the responsibility for shaping public health policies.

Sorano (Father of Obstetrics)

Sorano of Ephesus (98 to 138 AD), who can be considered the father of Gynecology and Obstetrics, studied and practiced medicine in Alexandria, then went to work in Rome during Hadrian's reign. There are those who consider it only inferior, in importance to the history of medicine, to Hippocrates and Galen[29].

He wrote a biography of doctors, and can therefore be considered the first author of a medical history.

His main work, *Gynaecia*, in 4 volumes, has two copies still preserved today, one of them in the Vatican library. It describes in detail the female genital tract and ways to prevent pregnancy, such as blocking the cervix with cotton, ointments or fatty substances. It presented several causes that could cause the interruption of menstruation, amenorrhea, and that could be a consequence from breastfeeding to genital infections. His work was written mainly for midwives.

He was the introducer of the delivery chair, which had armrests and buttocks and a crescent-shaped opening. He recommended certain procedures for difficult deliveries, especially in cases where the umbilical cord appears before the fetus.

It also details the way of conducting the delivery in abnormal presentations of the fetus, including what is considered its greatest contribution, or the podalic version. In this type of conduct, he recommends that the midwife, or the doctor who assists the pregnant woman, gently move the fetus inside the womb with the help of her hand so that the feet come out before the rest of the body.

He also described how to deal with the possible complications of childbirth, and also addressed topics related to Neonatology and Pediatrics.

Galen ("The prince of doctors")

No one exerted a greater influence on medicine than Claudius Galen, or Galen, a Greek physician who lived from AD 129 to 200. He wrote almost two hundred medical texts, systematizing all knowledge of Greek-Roman medical literature. His scientific production was so great that it was impossible to read or teach it during the training period of a professional.

The son of an architect, he was born in Pergamos, at the time the largest cultural center in Asia Minor and where there was a famous temple of Asclepius.

For nine years he studied medicine and philosophy in Somyrna, Corinth and Alexandria. Then he returned to his hometown and became a gladiator's doctor.

After four years he went to Rome, where he received greater recognition for his work. He was a physician to the emperor Marco Aurélio and, after his death, in 180, he became an adviser to Comodo, and later a physician to the emperor Sétimo Severo, who survived Galen.

He was a follower of the hypocratic school's theory of moods, and expanded it by classifying temperaments into four types:

1. Phlegmatic - related to phlegm or mucus; lazy, frivolous people; also related to water (among the four elements). Later, in the Middle Ages, astrology related these

people to the signs of fish, aquarium and capricorn.
2. Melancholic - related to black bile; stubborn, obstinate people; related to land. In astrology they correspond to the signs of Sagittarius, Scorpio and Libra.
3. Cholerics - related to yellow bile; audacious, exuberant people; related to air. In astrology they correspond to the signs of Virgo, Leo and Cancer.
4. Blood - related to blood; serene, peaceful people; related to fire. In astrology they correspond to the signs of Gemini, Taurus and Aries.

Galen was extremely vain, and the following sentence is attributed to him: "I did for medicine what Emperor Trajan did for the Roman Empire: I opened roads, built bridges. I am the sole creator of the true method of treating disease."

And yet, "I have never, until the present, made any mistake, either in the treatment or in the prognosis, as has happened to many other doctors of great reputation. If someone wants to achieve renown, the only thing they need to do is accept what I have been able to demonstrate".

Its therapeutic activity was based on the theory of opposites: it applied heat if the disease had been caused by the cold, or purgatives if it was the result of some excess food. He was also proficient in the use of medicines, which he himself produced.

Due to the fact that he performed anatomy studies only on animals, his work contained some false assumptions, as in relation to internal organs. He did, however, have a great deal of knowledge of physiology largely thanks to his experimental studies, done on animals.

A diagnosis he made on a Persian patient who complained of loss of sensation in the fingers of one hand is famous. Through a well-done medical history, Galen discovered that the case was due to an injury to the seventh cervical vertebra, resulting from the patient falling on a stone, an episode that only caused a momentary pain and was soon forgotten. He recommended bed rest and the application of a comforting plaster and the patient was cured.

Galen declared that any change in the function of the organism resulted from some type of injury, and that any injury led to some type of functional change, which is still true today.

It was probably the first to produce brain lesions in animals to distinguish between lesions of the brain lobes and those related to the brain stem and cerebellum. He recognized seven of the twelve cranial nerve pairs and distinguished between motor and sensitive nerves.

After Galen's death, an attempt was made to order and structure his teachings in order to create a coherent system, capable of disseminating his knowledge to medical students within a reasonable period of time. This was achieved around the 6th century AD, when, in Alexandria, several scholars of Galen's work managed to summarize it in 16 books, with four parts: the first, an introduction (books 1 to 4), the second dedicated to physiology (books 5 to 8), the third to pathology (books 9 to 14) and the fourth to therapy and hygiene (books 15 and 16).

His influence lasted for almost fifteen centuries, in part, probably, because his work coincided with various positions of Christianity. For Galen, everything was determined by a wise God and everything was a reflection of his perfection, and that perfection could be perceived in the human body. Galen's influence only diminished when Vesalius, in the 16th century, changed the study of anatomy entirely.

Eurico de Aguiar

The decline of Rome and the rise of religious civilizations

There were several causes of the decline of the Greco-Roman world, which was accentuated by the move of Emperor Constantine to Byzantium, in 330 AD According to some historians, imperialism was the main cause of the fall of Roman civilization. The enormous size of the territory conquered by Rome made the empire difficult to manage.

Other causes cited are the strong moral decay of society, which led to widespread corruption especially among the ruling classes and even within the army, in addition to great oppression of minorities and widespread poverty of the population.

There was also a great deal of permissiveness, with 32,000 prostitutes in Rome during Trajan's reign, and a liberation of customs. At the Coliseum, gladiators fought to the death, with a regrettable taste for cruelty developed among the people.

Due to the growth of Rome and other cities in the empire, with large crowds of people, several epidemics occurred, which contributed to further weaken the already weakened Roman power. In 166, there was an epidemic of exanthematic typhus. In 251, of smallpox. In the year 543, in the reign of Justinian, there was an epidemic of bubonic plague, which also caused thousands of deaths.

In face of all this, there was fertile ground for the emergence of a new civilization based on new ethical and moral values. It was from this moment that the preaching of Jesus Christ emerged and, with him, what at the beginning was only a sect, became in a few years a religion of enormous popular appeal.

It is important to emphasize that this new doctrine emerged as a synthesis of Christianity, Judaism and Hellenism, being addressed to all men and not to a particular people as was common to other religions of the time.

With Theodosius it became the official state religion[30], which was partly due to the fact that a large proportion of Roman soldiers were already Christians at the time. There are those who say that Emperor Constantine was converted in 315, after having seen, in the sky, a burning cross with the words "With this symbol you will win"[31], when returning from Gaul to face rivals who claimed the throne of Rome.

Islam emerged as a way to unite the Arab people around a religion and a common cause, through the preaching of Muhammad, in the early seventh century. His teachings are contained in the Koran, where the revelation of God was made to the prophet by the angel Gabriel, over twenty-three years, according to tradition.

According to Muhammad, "education is the duty of all Muslims, men, women, old people and children." And he still said, "seek Science, from the cradle to the grave. Seek Science, even if it is in China."

Inspired by the Jewish and Christian religion, Islam is monotheistic, believes only in Allah, induces the practice of charity and forgiveness among people, in addition to prohibiting the consumption of alcoholic beverages and pork.

He preaches fasting during the day, in the holy month of Ramadan, the practice of prayer five times a day, and the pilgrimage to his holy city, Mecca, at least once in his life.

Muhammad was not only the founder of a religion, but also of an Arab state, based in Medina. It was the duty of the faithful to conquer as much of the world as possible from Islam.

After Muhammad's death in 632, a great wave of Saracen expansion spread across Asia, Africa and Europe. About a hundred years after the death of the prophet of Islam, half the civilized world was dominated by Muslims. This empire was conquered without major struggles, more because of the fragility presented by the enemies than by the great supremacy of the Arab armies.

This expansion motivated the crusades, from 1096 to 1272, a religious war whose emblem was to recover the city of Jerusalem for Christians, but which in fact aimed to regain the lost territories for the Arabs.

While the influence of Christianity in Western Europe was predominant, between the 5th and 9th centuries, Islam reached its peak between the 7th and 13th centuries.

Art and Cure

The decline in the importance of the art of healing

The Middle Ages last for about a thousand years, or, more precisely, it is delimited between the division of the Roman Empire into the Roman Empire of the West and the East, in 395, and the fall of Constantinople in 1453, by the Ottoman Turks. In its first half, there was a setback in society's attitude towards rationalism, especially between the 10th and 11th centuries.

The medieval man's mind was turned to death, which had become a collective obsession. The symbol of death was found in many places, from graves to rings and home ornaments.

The disease was again seen as a punishment or punishment, or as a result of demonic possessions. As a result, people resorted to magic rituals or prayers, and the practice of medicine entered a long period of discredit and discredit.

Saint Augustine, who lived from 354 to 430, contributed to this view when he said: "all the illnesses of Christians must be attributed to demons and, in a special way, to those who torment the newly baptized; yes, even newborn babies, entirely without guilt".

On the other hand, the fact that the cities of the time were true human settlements, with precarious hygiene conditions, the lack of an adequate system of water and sewage networks and the lack of a waste removal routine, with a consequent increase of the population of rats and insects, contributed to infectious diseases occurring frequently, and not infrequently, in an epidemic.

The precariousness of medicine at the time, which could do little against different outbreaks, as in the epidemics of typhus, bubonic plague, smallpox, diphtheria, malaria, typhoid, dysentery, in addition to leprosy (now known as leprosy), which was very frequent, contributed significantly to the loss of credibility in medical practice.

The black plague alone, in 1347 and 1348, eliminated around 25 million people in Europe, and in some places the population was reduced by up to 75%.

Art of healing and Christianity

With the expansion of Christianity, from the beginning of the Middle Ages, and the renewed association between disease and sin, nothing could be more natural than that the Catholic Church was constantly present in the treatment and care offered to the sick. The Bible is rich in healing quotes made by Jesus Christ, in addition to the physical reparation being accompanied by the expulsion of demons or other "impure spirits".

As a result, the Church has increasingly taken on health care, since Christianity preached fraternity and charity to the humble and afflicted, in addition to considering suffering as a blessing for the salvation of the soul.

In addition, with a considerable distance from what was happening in the real world, Christianity led many of its followers to a greater indifference to the accumulation of goods in this world, which also contributed to their lesser participation in the economic activities of European countries.

Or, as Weatherford wrote[32], "for most of human life, religion used stories and rituals to arouse emotions such as fear of the unknown, eagerness to seek the invisible, to live forever or some other product that could not previously be obtained on earth".

On the other hand, in times of bloody conflict, no one could find the peace and calm needed to care for patients outside religious orders.

Hospitals emerged as Christian institutions. St. Helena, mother of Emperor Constantine, founded a hospital in the year 330, after moving the capital from the Roman Empire to Byzantium, which would later change its name to Constantinople. In 369, a hospital was created in Caesarea, by St. Basil, for the needy population.

Because of their own life of recollection and study, Benedictine monks ended up taking over medical care in the Western world for more than five centuries. This period of history is called the period of monastic medicine.

The founder of the Benedictine order, Benedicto de Nursia, from Montecassino, strongly influenced his monks to care for the sick. One of the first members of this community, Cassiodorus (490 to 575), who had been minister of Theodoric (king of one of the Germanic peoples who ruled Rome), and who later joined the Benedictine order, recommended the study of medicinal plants and the works of old doctors. With the missionary monks, medicine was infiltrating the peoples who adopted Christianity.

Eurico de Aguiar

In 805, Benedictines began to receive medical instruction as part of their formal apprenticeship, under the name of physics, and the doctors so trained were called physicists.

Most medicines were made by the monks themselves, from plants that they cultivated themselves. In each monastery there was a botanical garden, where the religious collected material for the preparation of their medicines, a pharmacy, a library and a place to treat the sick. In libraries, monks translated classic Greek texts into Latin.

The holy houses of mercy have spread throughout the world, with various religious orders taking over the treatment of the poor.

In France, hospitals were known as Hôtel-Dieu. The first appeared in Lyon, in 542. The one in Paris, founded in the 7th century, by the city's bishop, S. Landry, had 1,200 beds, only half of which with individual beds. The others received three to five patients per bed. Hospitals were run entirely by religious orders.

Lay medicine, despite continuing to exist, entered a phase of decline, only to regain part of its prestige after the emergence of European universities, from the 12th century onwards.

The decline of monastic medicine reached its peak in the 11th century. His success took the monks farther and farther from the monasteries and their religious obligations.

Many began to earn a lot of money from the activity and forgot about charity when it came to treating the poorest sick. Various Church councils were gradually restricting these medical activities, until their complete prohibition.

With the Council of Tours in 1163 (The Church does not spill blood), the Church prohibited monks from performing surgery. With this, it was no longer the doctors' responsibility, since most of them were religious. The surgery was then carried out only by barbers and charlatans of all kinds.

New religious orders have also emerged, such as the Dominicans and the Franciscans, clearly hostile to participation in scientific activities.

Paulus of Aegina

Considered as one of the greatest doctors of all time, he lived in the 7th century and studied in Constantinople and Alexandria. He published a collection of seven books on different topics, the most important of which is about surgery. In it, it addressed the treatment of uterine and breast cancer, in addition to the lithotomy technique, castration, treatment of gynecological lesions, and anal fistulas, hemorrhoids and fractures. He was also the creator of a system for bladder irrigation, using an ox bladder connected to a catheter, which would be a precursor system to the current bladder catheter.

The Arabs

"In medicine, absolute truth is an objective that cannot be achieved, and everything written in books is worth less than the experience of a sensible doctor." This phrase is from Abu Bakr Muhammad ibn-Zakasiya al-Razi, better known as

Rhazes, one of the most important Arab doctors, who lived from 860 to 932.

The aphorism is part of the book *Liber medicinalis ad almansorem*, which Rhazes wrote based on several texts from the ancient Greeks. In another of his books, *Liber de pestilentia*, accurately describes diseases such as measles and chickenpox.

Contrary to all types of quackery, Rhazes fought the excessive importance given to examining patients' urine.

At the time, doctors were absurd to believe until the examination of this material was sufficient to make the diagnosis of diseases, even without the presence of their clients.

Avicenna or Abu Ali al-Husayn Ibn Sina, who lived from 980 to 1037, is considered the greatest Arab physician of the Middle Ages. He was extremely intelligent, and at the age of ten he knew the entire Koran, the holy book of Islam.

At 18, he was already considered an experienced doctor and, after curing the prince of Bukhara, of a serious illness, he was rewarded with unrestricted access to his library.

He wrote a fundamental work, *Al Schafa*, a true philosophical encyclopedia, in which he sought to reconcile Neoplatonic ideas with Aristotelian doctrines.

His political views had aristocratic content. The rulers, according to Avicenna, are the great loners who, due to their isolation, are better able to reach universal reason.

His main medical work, *Canon*, served as a reference text in the western world until the 17th century. Avicenna was also a great admirer of the ancient Greek doctors, and his books remained true to their main teachings.

Abdallitif of Baghdad (1161–1231) was the first physician to find errors in Galen's work. He had the opportunity to examine thousands of skeletons, especially those who died of hunger and epidemics, then frequent in Egypt, where he went to visit Maimonides, another great Arab doctor.

Among Abdallitif's discoveries, which convinced him of the advantages of personal investigation instead of the knowledge acquired through the books of the time, that the jaw was a single bone, rather than formed by several pieces, as Galen proclaimed.

Maimonides was an Arab of Jewish origin, born in Cordoba, who lived from 1135 to 1204. He wrote a treatise, Astonished Guide, where he tries to reconcile faith with reason, presenting a negative theology according to which man can only know God indirectly, that is, for what He is not, a thesis that exerted considerable influence in medieval Christian philosophy.

He was many centuries ahead of his time, both in philosophy and in his view of medicine. He believed in a healthy mind in a healthy body, in the healing powers of nature, in the values of diet, rest, exercise, and simple remedies. Like Moses, he also wrote about hygiene.

The Arabs were largely responsible for the development of chemistry, having produced new medicines thanks to the advances they achieved in the field of pharmacology and the development of methods initially used by alchemists, such as crystallization, sublimation and distillation of substances.

According to Muslims, the seven celestial bodies they knew (Sun, Moon, Mercury, Mars, Venus, Jupiter and Saturn) corresponded to the seven days of the week and the seven metals, that is, gold, silver, iron, mercury, tin, lead and copper. Under the influence of the planets, these metals were born on earth from a common substance, the philosopher's stone.

Alchemists tried to discover the secret of this phenomenon, so that they could convert iron or lead into gold. They also said that drinking gold meant drinking the elixir of life, which was the secret of eternal youth or eternal life.

Nicholas Flamel, considered the most important alchemist of the 14th century, invested a large part of his life in the search for alchemical transformations that would allow him to come to find the philosopher's stone.

In addition, he was very interested in the occult. He believed in crystallomancy, that is, in the ability to see the future through the production of images reflected in shiny objects.

Another Flamel contemporary, John Dee, thought that the key to transmuting common metals for the development of the philosopher's stone could occur through angelic messages obtained through crystallomancy.

Finally, it can be said that many dedicated their lives and committed their fortunes in the search for the philosopher's stone. Although they never found it, some ended up discovering several chemical substances of great use, which are still widely used today.

The first universities

The word *university* comes from Latin and means *the whole*, since in these institutions there was a claim to contain all existing human knowledge.

Although there is one or another isolated faculty, such as medicine, in Montpellier, founded in the 9th century; that of Salerno (in southern Italy), created in the 10th century, and that of law, in Bologna, created in the 11th century, universities emerged in the 12th and 13th centuries, as a result of the growth and wealth of medieval European cities.

The Salerno school emerged next to a hospital founded by the Benedictines in the 7th century, that is, it was a consequence of monastic medicine.

Bologna was the first university to be created, around 1180, and since 1156 it already had a well-structured medical school.

The teaching was eminently theoretical, which resulted in the training of a few doctors with some practical experience, especially regarding surgery.

The first autopsies performed in Bologna took place at the end of the 13th century. The sections were commanded by a teacher, who from his chair (a large raised structure, with steps and a reading table) commanded the class, while a younger colleague, *ostensor*, pointed the incision line and a subordinate employee, *demonstrator*, performed the dissection.

Even with the possible permission of dissections by order of magistrates, as in cases of suspected poisoning, it was not until 1482 that Pope Sixtus IV - Pope from 1471 to 1484 - issued a bull allowing practice on human corpses. As a result, he came to promote the development of anatomy in European universities, as in Bologna, Padua, Paris and Montpellier. With this, the teaching of surgery took a new impulse in medical schools.

During this period, medical schools in Italian cities were the most prestigious in the world and between the 12th and 15th centuries several universities were created in France, Germany, England, Holland and Scandinavia.

An interesting fact of this period was the fact that both teachers and students came from different places and countries, but as the universal language of the cultured world was Latin, everyone understood each other perfectly.

Astrology and diseases

In all civilizations, and particularly among the oldest, the movements of the sun, the earth and the stars have always fascinated humanity.

For the ancient Egyptians, a new sun was created each day, reached its peak at noon and died in twilight.

In an ancient papyrus the earth is represented as a lying figure, covered with leaves, and the shimmering body of a celestial goddess spreading over it, carrying two boats, one to take the rising sun and the other to take the setting sun.

Representations of the land as a great plain, above which the firmament rested, appear in stories of Hindus, Greeks and several other peoples.

Above the earth were the clouds and the brightness of the stars at night was provided by paradise, which was beyond the clouds.

This idea of a flat land with paradise on top persisted for many centuries, until Pythagoras maintained that it was spherical. The prevailing view, however, was of a land with different geometric shapes[33].

The ancient Hindus believed in a hemispheric land, supported by four elephants standing on a huge turtle floating in a universal ocean.

Whatever form was admitted to our planet, there was great concern about how it was supported.

Some thought it floated in the water, others thought it had roots, or that it rested on twelve pillars, and that only through sacrifices would the pillars remain upright.

Some still thought that the earth was shaped like an egg, that it floated in water and that it was surrounded by fire.

Several ancient peoples observed that different groups of stars, or constellations, were close to the sun at dawn and dusk, at different times of the year.

A certain group of stars could be close to sunrise in one month, and could be above it or not be seen in the next month.

Thus, a constellation was associated with each month, and twelve groups of stars or constellations would form the zodiac.

The groups of stars high above the sun at dawn and dusk were used as a kind of celestial compass and the sun would take a year to complete its journey through paradise.

The division of the zodiac into twelve signs was used by different peoples, such as the Chaldeans, Egyptians, Hindus, Persians, Greeks and Romans.

The sign of aries is the first in the order because it is the constellation that coincides with the spring equinox in the northern hemisphere, when the duration of the days and nights is the same.

Astrology corresponds to the art of predicting or determining the influence of planets and stars on human affairs.

The etymological origin comes from the Greek words *astron* (star) and *logos* (spoken word, speech), which would correspond to the language of the stars.

Since the Mesopotamians, there is a strong association between astrology and health, that is, the position of the different stars and constellations in the sky, in each period of the year, it would act on us making us more or less vulnerable to certain diseases.

As already mentioned, this idea of the Babylonians was initially related to the influence of the moon on the movements of the tides.

In India astrology and medicine have evolved together since the most remote times and the highly advanced knowledge related to astrology and medicine is preserved in Indian sacred scriptures that have been passed down from generation to generation.[34].

Due to the fact that both astrology and medicine developed from a common axis, astrological principles related to prevention, health care and disease relief were applied as rituals, or even as part of religious ceremonies.

A student of the stars gave guidance on how to take the medication at the most appropriate time so that it would have the best effect to alleviate the sufferer's suffering.

Then, from the humoral theory, the body being made up of moods, that is, organic liquids, it came to believe that the moods of the human body should also be influenced by the stars.

Returning to Galen, we remember that people related to phlegm or mucus would be associated with the signs of fish, aquarium and capricorn, and their temperament would be of the phlegmatic type.

Those related to black bile, on the other hand, would be associated with the signs of sagittarius, scorpion and libra, with their melancholic temperament.

Choleric temperaments would be related to yellow bile and the signs of virgin, lion and cancer.

And finally, those with blood temperament would relate to the signs of twins, bull and Aries.

However, one of the most important texts that is still a reference in astrology today is the *Tetrabiblos*, written by Claudius Ptolemy, in Alexandria in the 2nd century AD[35]

Under the influence of some Greek philosophers, such as Plato and Aristotle, Ptolemy wrote two works of great significance for the West: the *Tetrabiblos* where he addresses astrology and *Almagest*, in which the geocentric theory is presented and becomes the astronomical paradigm until become overtaken by the works of Copernicus and Galileo.

His distinction between astronomy and astrology was as follows: the first is science that deals with the movements of celestial bodies, which are regular, immutable and perfect; the second, on the other hand, deals with the changes that the movements of celestial bodies cause in earthly things.

According to Ptolemy, making a person's horoscope constituted what we now call an astrological chart and for its realization it was necessary to support some personal data, such as date of birth, in addition to the place and time.

From there, the scenario of what would be happening in the sky at that moment in which the person was born would be defined, that is, for astrology this unforgettable moment marks the beginning of the person's presence in the world and from there a trend is traced of what may come to happen to her in the future.

This tendency, however, was not fatalistic or deterministic, as Ptolemy himself acknowledged. Throughout life, other factors may arise, such as different types of education and life habits and situations, which may change the trend initially presented.

For Ptolemy, astrology would serve for the prevention and

preparation of the spirit for the situations that may occur, also saying that, on earthly things, there are interferences from other causes, besides the celestial ones, such as luck, the environment and others that can oppose what was previously written in the stars.

In the realization of the astrological chart, the celestial space is divided into twelve signs, beginning with that of the ram, and the terrestrial space is also divided into twelve houses, with the ascendant corresponding to the cusp of the first house.

Each house would be associated with a sector of life, such as work, health, marriage, family, children and money.

Ptolemy also established familiarities between planets and signs, defined by the figure of the triangle, since the equilateral triangle is the geometric shape that presents more harmony:

- Aries, Leo and Sagittarius, signs governed by the Sun and Jupiter, and which correspond to the triangle of fire.

- Taurus, Virgo and Capricorn, signs governed by Venus and Moon, and which correspond to the triangle of the earth.

- Gemini, Libra and Aquarius, signs governed by Saturn and Mercury, and which would correspond to the triangle of air.

- Cancer, Scorpio and Pisces, signs ruled by Mars, which would correspond to the water triangle.

According to Ptolemy, each star would have dominion over certain parts of the organism or function, such as[36]:

- Saturn: right ear, spleen, bladder, mucus and bones.

- Jupiter: lungs, arteries, semen and touch.

- Mars: left ear, kidneys, veins and genitals.

- Sun: brain, heart, tendons, parts of the right side and vision.

- Venus: liver, muscles and smell.

- Mercury: tongue, bile, buttocks, speech and thought.

- Moon: stomach, belly, uterus, left side parts and swallowing.

Still in his book, Ptolemy refers to the relationship between comets, conditions of the moon and stars and events that could occur on our planet.

This influenced many people, making several epidemics throughout history justified as being due to the influence of the stars.

Bubonic plague, which decimated a large part of the European population in the 14th century, was considered to have been caused by the conjunction of the planets Saturn, Jupiter and Mars on March 24, 1345.

An influenza epidemic that occurred in London in 1510 was related to the appearance of comets, four years earlier[37].

The cholera pandemic, which started in 1817, was related to the phases of the moon and also as an omen of the appearance of Halley's comet in 1835.

In turn, meteors announced that new epidemics would soon emerge, that is, the human spirit always sought to relate celestial phenomena as a harbinger of new epidemics or new natural disasters.

This is perfectly understandable by the fact that, until today, astrologers and their predictions continue to exercise considerable fascination and influence over several people from the most diverse strata of society.

Physiotherapy

Among the various modalities of physiotherapy, hydrotherapy, and, in particular, baths in hydro-mineral estates have been used since the most remote times.

In ancient Greece, the temples of Asclepius were built near water sources with healing properties.

The Romans were aware of the therapeutic virtues of water and also used hydrotherapy regularly.

In the Middle Ages, Montecatini and Karlsbad waters were the most popular.

Therapy based on sea water, which comes from ancient Rome, where it was indicated for cases of tuberculosis, still leads thousands of bathers today to frequent several summer resorts on the coast of several countries.

Massages were also widely used since antiquity, and Greeks and Romans gave them great importance as a therapeutic weapon.

Massages and passive movement of the limbs, especially after fractures, have become widely used over time.

Gymnastic exercises have also started since antiquity. In the 18th century, gymnastics was indicated as a way to acquire control over the will over movements and in opposition to the tendency to relax the body.

Thermotherapy was used in conjunction with hydrotherapy, and currently using infrared rays.

Amerindians and diseases

It is estimated that the Indians of America are descendants of Asian peoples, who would have crossed the Behring Strait twelve thousand years ago, and then dispersed throughout the continent.

Although some believe that pre-Columbian America was not completely isolated from Europe until the 15th century (there is evidence that the Vikings here were around 1000), it is likely that syphilis is a disease originating in the New World. The most modern findings of paleopathology, an area of knowledge that studies diseases through archaeological evidence, suggest that endemic syphilis affected North American Amerindian populations well before Columbus's arrival in 1492.

According to Braudel[38], " syphilis expands from the discovery of pre-Columbian America: it is an offer, revenge, some said of the losers. Of the four or five theories that doctors today support, the most likely is perhaps the one that makes the disease a creation, or rather, a recreation originating in the sexual relations between two races (influence of Treponema pertinens on Treponema pallidum). In any case, the evil turns out to be terrible in Barcelona after Colombo's return parties (1493), then it spreads at a galloping pace; it is an endemic, rapid, deadly disease. In four or five years he goes around Europe, moves from country to country with illusory names:

mal-de-Naples, mal-french, *the french disease* or *lo malo francioso* ; France, given its geographical position, wins this vocabulary war ".

When Cabral arrived in South America in1500, there were about four million Indians in the territory.

Cabral would not have been the first to arrive here, according to documents that report the passage of another Portuguese navigator, Duarte Pacheco, in 1498, who would have landed at a point near the border between Maranhão and Pará, and who later would have gone to the island of Marajó and known at the mouth of the Amazon River. His findings were not disclosed because, according to the Tordesillas Treaty, this territory would belong to Spain.

According to Del Priore and Venancio[39] , the Frenchman Jean Cousin was at the mouth of the Amazon in 1488 and the Spanish Diogo de Lepe and Alonso de Hojeda would also have passed through stretches of the north coast of our lands before 1500.

Shortly after the arrival of the Portuguese, a good part of the indigenous population was decimated, mainly by the diseases brought by white men. The Indians did not have immunity to viruses such as measles and smallpox, which are easily and quickly spread.

Today this great susceptibility of our Indians to the new diseases brought from Europe is explained not as some kind of disability, but as a consequence of the Amerindian populations being biologically very homogeneous from the genetic point of view.

Because they never had contact with these microbes, they did not develop the immunity necessary for their survival.

The art of healing of the Aztecs, Mayans and Incas

Both the Aztecs and the Maya - people who lived in the territory that today corresponds to Mexico, Guatemala and Honduras - added little to what we know today. It was a primitive medicine, with a strong content of mysticism. Quite impregnated with magic, more linked to witchcraft and beliefs and little different from that of other primitive peoples of America.

Tobacco was considered a plant capable of curing various diseases. It was used as smoke, chewed or even inhaled as snuff.

The Incas, who occupied a large part of the Andean territory, showed a higher level of development in the health area.

People with disabilities, widows and the elderly were protected by the state, which represented a major step forward in terms of social policy.

Pieces of land were reserved so that these people could be maintained. In addition, the disabled - deaf, dumb, blind, paralyzed and those with congenital diseases - were given simpler functions and for which they were trained, such as security guard jobs, doormen and domestic servants.

Among the drugs used by the Incas, the main ones include coca and the bark of a tree called "cinchona", from which quinine, a potent antimalarial, was later extracted and which is still used today.

Most important diseases in the Middle Ages

Leprosy

The man in whose skin or flesh appears a strange color, a tumor or a kind of shiny spot, which is an indication of leprosy disease, will be taken to Priest Aaron or any of his children, who, if he sees leprosy on his skin, with his hair whitened and the part that looks like a leper more depressed than the remaining skin, will declare that it is leprosy sore and will consider it impure, and what has it will be separated from the company of others. His clothes will be torn, his head disheveled, he will cover himself up to his mustache and scream: impure, impure! As long as he is leprous and unclean, he will live alone, outside the village.

Leviticus 13, 2-3; 45-46

Leprosy represented the great plague of the Middle Ages, causing more panic and fear than any other disease. In fact, the term was used to frame a series of pathologies with repercussions on the skin, ranging from non-infectious diseases, such as eczema and psoriasis, to smallpox or even syphilis in its secondary phase.

With the return of the Crusaders to their cities of origin, many brought disease, and leprosy, being endemic among the poor population, reached epidemic proportions in the 13th and 14th centuries.

The leprosy patient was totally discriminated against, considered impure, being forced to be totally ostracized and, even before his death occurred, society had him as dead and deprived of all civil rights. When he walked, he carried a rattle to warn the others of his arrival, in order to prevent them from any contagion.

The Catholic Church took on the task of fighting leprosy to facilitate the isolation of the sick, having created several leprosariums since the 6th century. They were called lazaretos because, initially, the sick were interned in the monasteries of S. Lázaro, in memory of the famous leper of the Bible.

In France alone, at the beginning of the 11th century, there were two thousand lazarets.

Only in 1874, the Norwegian physician and botanist Gerhard Henrik Hansen began the process of demythologizing the disease by identifying its etiological agent, Mycobacterium leprae.

From then on, leprosy started to be seen as a divine punishment and started to be seen as it really is, that is, a relevant public health problem, especially in the poorest regions of the world, such as in central Africa, in the north of the country. Brazil and India.

The Black Death

Two pandemics of bubonic plague hit the world in the Middle Ages. The first in the reign of Justinian, of the Eastern Roman Empire, in 542 and 543, and the second that reached practically the whole of Europe in 1347 and 1348, considered the one that caused more deaths at all times. In it, half the population of London died. Unmanned ships roamed the North Sea and the Mediterranean, spreading the infection when they reached the beaches.

In *Decameron*, in 1353, Boccaccio described the dantesque scenes he witnessed: "The condition of people was unfortunate to describe. They got sick by the thousands daily and died without being attended to or rescued. Many died on the streets; others died in their homes, and this was only known from the stench they gave off from their decomposing bodies. Since there are no more places in the cemeteries to bury so many bodies, they were stacked by the hundreds in large ditches, like ship goods, and then covered with a little bit of earth".

The probable origin of this latest pandemic may be linked to wild rodents from Central Asia, where there is a reservoir of this disease, or the presence of wild animals carrying the plague agent. Hence the disease went to Italy and France, and to Germany, then reaching Russia. Ships were of great importance in bringing the disease to several countries, causing the disease to spread rapidly.

According Braudel[40], "the plague's enormous archive never ceases to increase, the explanations of huddling together. To begin with, the disease is at least double: pulmonary plague on the one hand, a new form of evil that erupts in history with the 1348 pandemic in Europe; bubonic plague, on the other hand, older (buboes that form in the groin and gangrene). They are the marks of God, *God's tokens* or, more correctly, *tokens* , in French the *tacs* , similar to the metal or leather buttons that traders put into circulation".

Many strange theories were developed to explain this epidemic. Some justified it by the conjunction of the planets Saturn, Jupiter and Mars on March 24, 1345, which would be the natural foreshadowing that a catastrophe would occur. Others said that the wells had been poisoned by Jews and lepers, which led many innocent people to be pursued and even killed at the stake, accused of witchcraft.

Because it is a bacterial disease transmitted through the flea of rats, it requires that hygienic conditions are precarious for its development. The human settlements that were the cities of the Middle Ages, in addition to the general lack of hygiene, fully favored the emergence of these infections.

Isolating patients was one of the rare alternatives tried to control the disease. If a person was affected in a home, the authorities were immediately notified. After being examined, and the infection found, the patients were kept in their homes and forced to isolate everyone who had contact with the patient. Through messengers, family members began to receive what they needed to survive.

The isolation period for patients and their contacts, which at the beginning was 14 days, was up to 40 days in Venice and other European cities. The term quarantine comes from this longer period of isolation.

The black death of the sea

With the great navigations, which began in the late 15th and early 16th centuries, a new disease arose that led sailors to death by hemorrhage. On long journeys, which took months, scurvy was a frequent and terrifying disease. He had previously wreaked havoc in besieged cities when the supply of supplies was cut.

On the voyage in which he discovered the sea route to the Indies, in 1498, Vasco da Gama lost fifty-five sailors due to the disease.

For more than a hundred years, scurvy has led many sailors to death, and was thus described by Camões[41]:

And it was, that of raw and ugly disease

The most I've never seen,

Many life, and in strange and alien land

The bones are forever buried.

Who will be without seeing him?

That so misshapenly inflated him

The gums in the growing mouth

The meat and rotted together

Rotting and a fetid and gross

Smell that the neighboring air infected;

They didn't have a cunning doctor there,

Subtle surgeon was least thought of;

But any in this craft little instruction

He cut through the rotten meat like this,

As if she had been killed, and well suited

Because whoever had it was dead.

In 1593, Admiral Richard Hawkins, through personal experience, relates that ten thousand sailors died from scurvy and that he, in his remarks, wrote that what I saw u, m ore hit for this disease, were oranges sorrel and lemons[42].

Later, already in 1601, an interesting experiment was made with an English fleet commanded by James Lancaster. Five ships left England for India.

On this trip, three teaspoons of lemon were administered every day to the men who served on the largest of the ships. When the fleet reached the Cape of Good Hope, there were already a large number of sailors with scurvy on the other four smaller ships who had not received lemon juice. There were no cases of the disease on the larger vessel. Despite the very evident results, this experience was not properly considered at the time.

However, the classic work on scurvy was published in 1753 by James Lind, a British naval surgeon, where he demonstrates that the disease could be eliminated as long as lemon juice was offered to sailors. Lind, through personal experience, proved the healing power of various products, such as watercress, tamarind, oranges and lemons.

However, despite all this evidence, s nly in 1795, a year after the death of Lind, the British Admiralty ordered during transoceanic travel all the sailors were given a daily allowance of lemon juice, which gave them an appropriate contribution of vitamin C, as is currently known.

Other medieval diseases

Some diseases were known in the Middle Ages with names that no longer exist. Others were known by more than one name or expression and would represent today not one, but a set of diseases, such as:

1. "St. Valentine's disease" or "badly expired" - would be

equivalent to epilepsy.
2. "Penitência de São Quirino" or "Vengeance of São João" - would be equivalent to tumors, varicose veins and boils.
3. "Fogo de Santo Antonio" - today it could be erysipelas, gangrene and even cholera.[43]
4. "Baile de São Vito" - a disease that arose in 1374, when many people started dancing like possessed neurotics. It is suspected that it may have been a picture of collective hysteria. There are authors who also attribute neurological causes to this disease, such as chorea and Parkinson's.

The empirical art of cure

Medicine consists of putting drugs that are not known in a body that is even less known. Voltaire

New philosophical ideas (16th and 17th centuries)

In the famous cave myth[44], Plato likens men to prisoners kept under irons, where they can only look in one direction. With a fire at his back, he considers his shadows as part of the real world. When one of the prisoners escapes and leaves, he finds the sunlight, he knows the truth and realizes that until then he had been deceived by his own imagination and reflects sadly on his long life in the darkness. He also recognizes that escaping the cave and its darkness, he reaches the light of truth and conscience. He then becomes a philosopher, as he is the one who has the true knowledge of reality.

After the long period of darkness in the Middle Ages, three philosophers were particularly important in encouraging scientific thought: Francis Bacon, René Descartes and John Locke. However, other thinkers were also essential to the development of a philosophy of modern science, as was the case with Hobbes, Hume, Pascal, Spinoza, Berkeley and Leibniz.

Bacon, lawyer, member of Parliament, creator of the phrase "knowledge is power", had in the book *The promotion of knowledge* his most important work.

The whole foundation of his philosophy was practical: through scientific discoveries and innovations, humanity could dominate the forces of nature and, from there, come to have a better life. This was in opposition to the Greeks, for whom science was an essentially speculative and less important task.

He was the first philosopher to emphasize the value of the inductive method, through which one can start from particular experience to generalizations and laws. He was also a pioneer in giving the scientific procedure a logical systematization.

He recommended writing down all known facts, and that all new observations and the results of new experiments be tabulated, so that the connection between the phenomena and their resulting general laws could be more easily manifested.

René Descartes, considered the founder of modern philosophy, is the author of the phrase "I think, therefore I am", the first principle of his philosophy. The knowledge of our own thoughts is the only fact that is absolutely true. This principle weakens what we perceive by the senses when compared to what we capture by reasoning.

His most important works were the *Discourse on Method* and *Meditations*. Its philosophy is based on methodical doubt, or on a methodical skepticism that could be presented as follows:

- Never accept as truth other than what I perceive as such.

- Divide each of the difficulties into as many parts as possible and as many as necessary to resolve them.

- Conduct my thoughts in order, starting with the simplest and easiest to be known objects, to climb, little by little, to the knowledge of the most complex.

- Make enumerations so complete and revisions so general that you are sure you have omitted nothing.

In his book *La Géometrie*, he made a considerable contribution to the evolution of mathematics, attributing to it the notation we use for equations, such as lower-case letters at the end of the alphabet (x, y, z) for unknown quantities and lower-case letters at the beginning of the alphabet (a, b, c) for known quantities, as well as exponents on a variable to indicate powers.

With the *Discourse on the Method*, he inaugurates epistemology, saying that reason or common sense, guided by the method, would be sufficient for access to the truth, and is no longer the privilege of a few elect.

With the creation of the scientific method[45], and as a result, with the creation of analytical tools, science and knowledge are now democratized and accessible to a greater number of people.

Although Descartes proposed that body and mind act separately, as an inference to his famous phrase "I think, therefore I am", and that as a consequence of this there would be a hierarchy between reason (linked to the brain) and emotions (linked to the soul), studies of neuroanatomy, neurophysiology and neuropsychology have shown that body and mind are closely linked, and that emotions and rationality are also related to the development of our thinking structure and how we manage to deal with the issues that affect our daily. Without emotions, reason does not develop properly, and also without reason, emotions can act contrary to social interest.

John Locke, one of the pioneers of philosophical liberalism, had as one of his striking characteristics the lack of dogmatism. According to him, the truth is difficult to ascertain and a prudent man will always defend his opinions with a certain margin of doubt, which is a reflection of the influence that Descartes' ideas had on him. His fundamental work, *An essay concerning human understanding*, published in 1690, systematically addresses the questions of the origin, essence and certainty of human knowledge.

Love of truth, according to Locke, is a very different thing from love of a particular doctrine proclaimed as truth.

Enthusiasm, oblivious to reason, places fantasies - rather than reason - in a man's brain.

Locke is considered the founder of empiricism, a doctrine according to which all our knowledge derives from experience, with the exception of logic and mathematics.

He condemned absolutism in every way, being considered the father of liberal political theory in the 17th and 18th centuries. He believed that if men were born equal, they should have equal rights, as well as those necessary for their survival, such as the right to work and property.

Both Bacon and Descartes and Locke were against scholasticism, a doctrine strongly influenced by the Church, which thus held philosophy hostage to theology throughout the Middle Ages, its main thinkers being St. Thomas Aquinas and St. Augustine and who said "the truth is more in what God reveals than in the conjectures of men who walk in the dark".

The philosophers of that period contributed significantly to build enlightenment, which shifted the center of interest and concerns about the destiny of the soul, in the other world, towards improving living conditions in the world in which we live.

From the ideas of the Enlightenment there was a review of the authoritarian state, in the countries where it exerted the greatest influence, such as in England, France and in the English colony from which the United States of America arose.

The Renaissance

What characterizes the period of history after the Middle Ages is the diminishing authority of the Church and the increasing authority of science.

This lesser influence of the Church had the contribution of Martin Luther (1483-1546) and Calvin (1509-1564), who created a new religion, Protestantism, which soon spread to several European countries.

Another remarkable fact was the creation of the mobile type of printing by Gutenberg, who printed the first book, a Bible, in 1453, in an edition of 150 copies. From then on, the dissemination of knowledge was greatly expanded, and more people were able to access the information.

At the beginning of the Italian Renaissance, science still plays a limited role, since opposition to the Church was focused on the values of classical Greco-Roman culture. Only after Copernicus, with the publication of his book *On the revolutions of the celestial spheres*, in 1543, science really began to produce profound changes in European society.

Born in Pisa in 1564, the son of a cultured but impoverished nobleman named Vincenzio Galilei, who wanted to make him a merchant, Galileo Galilei started studying medicine at the age of 17, a course he did not complete. His greatest interest was investigations and mathematical studies.

In 1589 he was invited to teach the discipline at the University of Pisa and, three years later, at the University of Padua, where he taught for 18 years.

It had the merit of introducing mathematical rationalism as the basis of scientific thought, in addition to having done several researches in the field of Mechanics, which would later be used by Newton.

Perfected the telescope[46] and through it he developed several astronomical studies. In 1609 he had already managed to develop a device with a 30-fold magnification, which allowed great advances in science.

He described the irregularity of the lunar surface, discovered more than 500 stars never seen before, observed that the Milky Way was made up of a large number of stars, discovered Jupiter's four satellites and also sunspots.

He published several books, including one in support of Copernicus' heliocentric theory.

His works became more dangerous because he published them in Italian[47], instead of Latin, as was customary at the time.

It contradicted the geocentric theory that, according to him, was based only on the allegories existing in the Scriptures. With this, he was pursued by the Holy Inquisition, having at the end of his life to retract himself to escape the bonfire.

In the sentence, published in 1633, he was declared a suspect of heresy, obliged to abjure the Copernican doctrine and sentenced to house arrest until he died in 1642.

Galileo was also important for the book *Il Saggiatore* (The Tester), published in 1623, where he writes as a true philosopher of science. It says that for philosophy to become science it must get rid of the domain of authority, that is, it defends freedom of thought and even that true philosophy must be based fundamentally on observation, reasoning and mathematics.

Over time, the human species has been moving from the center to the periphery of the universe. Today, when we know that we are part of just one galaxy - with three hundred billion stars in its interior -, among billions of others existing in the universe, it is that we realize the real importance of human beings, which contradicts significantly the initial conception, when Ptolemy's ideas predominated.

In the arts, exponents of the Renaissance are the Italians Michelangelo (1475-1564), Leonardo da Vinci (1452-1519) and Raphaello (1483-1521), who went on to dissect dozens of corpses to better understand human anatomy and thus perfect his technique, creating works of extraordinary beauty. Besides them, the Venetians Titian, Tintoretto and Veronese were also very important.

Giorgio Vasari (1511 to 1574), a notable critic and art historian, in addition to being an architect and painter, published in 1550 the book *The lives of the best painters, sculptors and architects* , where he quotes Florentine Antonio Pollaiuolo (1432 to 1498) as one of first artists to dissect the human body. His most important work was the painting "O Martírio de S. Sebastião", where the results of this anatomical research are clearly demonstrated.

In the arts, the Renaissance received the name of naturalism.

Leonardo da Vinci left a considerable collection of works

with anatomical studies. He is still regarded today as one of the greatest anatomists of all time. In the book written about Leonardo, White[48] presents several drawings by the artist, such as studies of the muscles of the hands and face, the arm and shoulder, the brain, the eye, etc.

Illegitimate son of a notary named Ser Piero, with a peasant woman named Caterina, Leonardo was born in a small Tuscan town called Vinci, and from an early age he had a remarkable abundance of talents, which led him to treat his artistic potential with some lightness.

He rarely completed a painting, in addition to being given to bold technical experiments. He said that a painter's first goal was to make a flat surface look like a raised body that protrudes from that same surface.

He is the author of the painting that is considered the most famous and valuable of all time, the Mona Lisa or La Gioconda, as it is best known in Italy. The work, currently on display at the Louvre museum in Paris, seeks to portray the third wife of the wealthy Tuscan merchant Francesco del Giocondo, named Lisa di Gherardini, who at the time was about 25 years old. Leonardo took three years to complete it (1503 to 1506).

Other famous paintings by Leonardo are Bacchus (1513), Saint John the Baptist (1508-1513), The Virgin and Child with Sant'Ana (1508-1510), the Lady with an Ermine (1488-1490), Ginevra de Benci (1475) and La Belle Ferronière (1495 to 1499).

Leonardo's refined technique can be found in everyone, such as the internal movement known as the *counterpoint* (model sitting in a position while the face looks in a different direction), the play of shadows, the somewhat hidden appearance, as if enveloped in fog and a certain suggestion of androgyny.

The Renaissance represents a time of renewal in the field of arts and sciences, and the spirit of freedom and criticism is now opposed to the principle of authority that was the rule until then.

Andreas Vesalius (The anatomy reformer)

The son of a family of doctors, Vesalius, whose name was Andreas Wytinck van Wesel, was born in 1514 in Brussels. He studied medicine in Paris, and later settled in Padua, where at the end of 1537 he was appointed professor. The works of Italian naturalists had an enormous influence on the development of their work.

In 1543, then 28 years old, he published the monumental anatomy treatise *De Humanis corporis fabrica* (on the construction of the human body), consisting of seven volumes and seven hundred pages, with hand-colored illustrations. It was the first comprehensive text on the subject and that breaks with tradition, demonstrating that Galen was wrong in several aspects, such as the structure of the heart, the path of the veins, the sternum bone, the liver, the bile duct, the uterus and other aspects of anatomy. The Greek doctor's studies were done on animals, while Vesalius had written his book on knowledge acquired through the dissection of human corpses.

Vesalius was an extremely educated man, having translated several works from the Greek, Arab and Hebrew classics.

As contradicting Galen was heresy, it was widely criticized by his contemporaries. Despite being a professor of medicine and anatomy in Padua, he became bored with so many and so groundless criticisms that he decided to abandon the chair and accepted the invitation to serve as a doctor for Emperor Carlos V, and after Philip II, of Spain.

Years later he recognized his merit and, from then on, he started to be considered as he really deserved, that is, as one of the most notable doctors in history.

In his work, it also proved to be a mistake to separate surgery from medicine.

It is said that he was condemned to death by the Inquisition, for having dissected a nobleman while still alive. Vesalius would have been wrong, and it was only too late that he realized that his heart was still beating. Through Philip II's interference, his sentence would have been replaced by a pilgrimage to Jerusalem.

After going to the Holy Land in 1564, the ship he was traveling sank on the island of Zante, Greece, where he ended up dying of hunger and thirst, after walking for three days in a desert land.

The anatomical amphitheaters

Public curiosity about dissections grew extraordinarily in the 16th century. The public was invited as if to go to a play, and solemn invitations were made to influential people.

Anatomical amphitheaters were built in some cities, such as in Padua, in 1545, and in Leipzig, in 1580.

Girolamo Fracastoro (Creator of the contagion theory)

The word syphilis was created by Fracastoro, in a famous poem entitled *Syphilis Sive Gallicus Morbus,* or Syphilis, the French evil. This work sought to attribute the appearance of the disease to the French, while they attributed it to the Italians.

Published in 1530, this long poem described the story of a shepherd, named Syphilis, who, by rendering divine honors to his king, offends Jupiter. The deity sends Apollo to the land, who punishes the pastor by inflicting the punishment of a new disease, for which there is no known cure.

Fracastoro was a professor at the University of Padua, lived from 1483 to 1553, and some say his interest in syphilis was a consequence of also having the disease.

Syphilis was first detected in Barcelona, the city where Columbus' sailors returned after the discovery of America. Today it is known that the disease comes from the New World.

Europe had very favorable conditions for the development of this new pandemic. In Venice alone, with a population of 300,000 people, there were 12,000 prostitutes.

In 1546 Fracastoro publishes his most important work, *De contagione et contagiosis morbis*, where he formulates theories that, surprisingly, come very close to the modern theory of germs that cause infections. This, at a time when there was still no knowledge of microbes, can be considered quite significant.

Fracastoro distinguished three types of contagion: one direct from person to person; a second, through objects or clothing contaminated by the patient; and a third, which would be transmitted over the air. He said that vehicles for these diseases would have the power to quickly reproduce them. His theories were only confirmed centuries later, with Pasteur and Koch.

Paracelsus (Genius or charlatan?)

"Medicine is not only a science, but also an art. It does not consist of composing pills, plasters and drugs of all kinds, it deals, on the contrary, with the processes of life, which must be understood before being guided. A powerful will can heal, in which case hesitation, or doubt, can lead to failure. The character of the doctor can act more powerfully on the sick than all the drugs used," said Phillippus Teophrastus von Hohenheim, better known as Paracelsus, a name he wanted to be called for his opposition to Celso and other doctors of antiquity.

Born in Switzerland in 1493, Paracelsus was one of the most

controversial scholars in history. His interest ranged from the occult sciences, magic, astrology and alchemy, to natural science.

He traveled to several places, having studied in Vienna, Cologne, Paris and Montpellier. He also lived in the Iberian peninsula, Pomerania, Poland, Lithuania and Russia.

More than a dozen books were written about his life and work, in several languages.

Due to the cures made by important personalities of the time, such as Erasmus of Rotterdam, he was invited to teach at the University of Basel, the oldest in Switzerland.

There, he scandalized everyone by making his first conference in German, instead of traditional Latin, in addition to violently criticizing the works of Galen and Avicenna, even burning some of his works in public.

His opinions, which deeply attacked the foundations of ancient medicine, in addition to the violence and impetuosity of his personality, produced so many enemies that his stay at the university became impossible.

After two years, Paracelsus had to leave Basel and return to his life as a wandering doctor.

With it, medicines made with chemicals were introduced into medicine and pharmacology began to make use of several new products.

He said that all medicines were based on four basic pillars: philosophy, astrology, alchemy and virtue.

An important contribution of Paracelsus, who did not have the appropriate repercussion at the time, was his perception of the power of ether as an anesthetic. He found that by adding the substance to the poultry feed, in order to make the feed sweeter, they fell into a deep sleep and later woke up without any damage. Only in the 19th century did ether start to be used as an anesthetic in surgeries.

Paracelsus believed that matter was made of sulfur, mercury and salt, but this was done in a symbolic sense. He believed in salt as an element indestructible by fire; in mercury, a fluid that was vaporized, but not destroyed by fire; and sulfur, both modified and destroyed by fire. These principles were contained in the "great mystery", from which the four main elements of life arose: water, fire, earth and air.

His interest in the occult can be assessed by the following text: "If my will is filled with hatred against someone, I need to express this feeling in some way. This will be done precisely through the body. Undoubtedly, if my will is too violent or burning, it may happen that my desire will pierce and hurt the spirit of the hated person. And I can also forcefully enclose it in an image that I can make of it, deforming and distorting it to my liking, thus also achieving the intention to torment my enemy".

However, he warned: "On the other hand, anyone who remains impregnated with hatred, never wanting good, can attract to himself all the evil desired by others. Because if the evil spell exists only with the permission of the spirit, it can happen that the images of the evil transform into diseases, such as fevers, epilepsies, strokes and others. For this reason, it is good not to mock these things."

He also said that "progress can only be based on experimentation, and on the conclusions that can be deduced from it".

Paracelsus died in 1541, probably of cancer, in Salzburg.

After his death, he continued to have several followers, especially in England and Germany, most of whom belonged to the Rosicrucian sect, which still exists today.

Jean Fernel (Continuer of Vesalius work)

Considered one of the great anatomists of the 16th century, he lived from 1497 to 1558. He was a physician of King Henry II, and had a passion for Astronomy. He was a professor of medicine in Paris, and contributed to the correction of some concepts of Galen.

Wrote *Universal Medicine*, divided into physiology, pathology and therapeutics. He was the first to describe the condition of appendicitis and to suggest the syphilitic origin of aortic artery aneurysms. He was also a pioneer in believing that gonorrhea and syphilis were distinct diseases.

He was opposed to astrology, unlike most doctors of his day.

Of a melancholy nature, Fernel died shortly after the death of his wife.

Ambroise Paré (The patron of military medicine)

Paré (1510 to 1590), as a military doctor, accompanied a great expeditionary force that King Francis I of France had sent to Italy in order to conquer Turin.

There were then several battles, with many wounded from all types of weapons, but mainly by firearms. At that time, it was believed that the wounds caused by these weapons were poisonous due to gunpowder, and that the best treatment for this was cauterization with boiling oil.

This practice caused soldiers great pain and suffering. Paré used it until, one night, the oil ran out and he was forced to replace it with a mixture of rose water, egg yolk and turpentine.

He was surprised when, upon awakening, he found that the patients treated with the mixture were doing very well, almost painlessly, while those treated with boiling oil, in addition to showing signs of inflammation in their wounds, complained of severe pain. From then on, Paré decided not to treat his patients in the cruel way that was usual until then.

Paré, son of a barber-surgeon, began his practice with his father. This professional category, inferior to that of university-trained surgeons, was responsible for the treatment of wounds, cauterization, puncture of abscesses, in addition to shaving their clients. They also bleed.

Despite not knowing the languages of the formal science of the time, or Greek and Latin, Paré came to become the greatest surgeon in France, having been a physician to four kings of his country (Henrique II, Francisco II, Carlos IX and Henrique III). He introduced the technique of ligation of the arteries to control bleeding, also abandoning, in this case, the use of heat to stop bleeding. He also reintroduced surgical correction for cleft lip, which had been forgotten since the Arabs. Abolished castration for the routine treatment of male hernias.

In 1561 he published the book *Universal Surgery*, where he presented new surgical techniques and instruments that he had developed throughout his professional practice.

One day, after curing an officer seriously wounded in battle, Paré humbly said, "I treated him and God healed him."

Johann Weyer (Founder of Modern Psychiatry)

In 1231 Pope Gregory IX ordered the Dominican order to persecute and eliminate heretics through the Inquisition. Permanent sections have been installed in all Catholic countries, with torture being their main means of investigation.

During the sixteenth century, with the increasing independence of higher-level institutions from control by the authorities, astrology hitherto strongly supported by physicians is no longer as widely considered.

However, in other segments of society, the belief in witches and their power reaches its highest level.

Thus, and even more threatened by the emergence of Protestantism, the Church published, in 1485, a book called *Malleus Maleficarum* (Hammer of Witches), made by two Dominican inquisitors, recognizing witches as their enemies, and detailing the steps why suspicious people should go through: arrest, interrogation, torture and execution.

The main target of the book was women, defined as beings inferior and impure by nature, considered by the authors as true instruments of the devil.

Because they believed that witches were accomplices to the devil, the inquisitors condemned them to death at the stake.

In 1563, the German physician Johann Weyer published a book, *De Praestigiis Daemonius* (On Witchcraft), where he maintains that these persecuted people were, in fact, poor ignorant citizens, who had lost emotional control, and their minds had deteriorated. This, in an age of so many and so frequent disturbances and calamities, was an understandable phenomenon to occur.

Weyer believed that confessions obtained through torture were a terrible mistake. He denied the possibility of transforming men into animals and that witches could fly on broomsticks, as was the belief at the time.

He also said that nightmares and possessions were due to anguish, apprehension or suggestion. Magic potions, witchcraft and beliefs could drive some people insane, but never succeed in achieving the desired magical purposes. The diabolical arts and their ghosts should not frighten anyone.

His book was a great success, despite the great risk he took in divulging these opinions, and certainly contributed to improve the mentality of many people who lived in his time.

Unfortunately, however, the witch hunt continued to be widely used, with its heyday occurring during the 1600s, decades after the publication of Weyer's book.

Fabrizio de Acquapendente (Discoverer of vein valves)

Disciple of Gabriel Fallopio - discoverer of the tubes of the female genital apparatus -, Fabrizio (1537 to 1619) succeeded his master as professor of surgery at the University of Padua, at the age of 28. He had a great passion for anatomy, having understood that only by mastering this subject could the surgeon operate successfully. In 1603 he published his most important work, *De Venarum Ostiolis*, where he described, for the first time, the valves of the veins. This finding demonstrated that blood only circulates in one direction, or in the direction of the heart. This discovery was fundamental for one of his students, the Englishman William Harvey, to come after a few years to describe the blood circulation.

Fabrizio died in 1619, poisoned by opponents envious of his great professional success, since throughout his life he received proof of recognition for the much he did for the development of science.

European transformations

With the discovery of America by Columbus, and the new

trade routes in the Atlantic and Indian Ocean, there was a substantial decrease in the economic importance of Italy's ports.

The power of the cities of Venice and Genoa began to decline, at the same time that Italian territory continued to be devastated by the invasion of soldiers from France, Germany and Spain, in addition to the rivalry between Italian cities having been relevant to increase their wear and tear. As a result, medical knowledge was interrupted in its rapidly growing process in that region of Europe.

In Germany, in addition to bloody religious disputes, the 30-year war helped to halt a development process that seemed to be extremely favorable to the German people.

In the same period, England and the Netherlands reached the height of their maritime power, resulting in reflexes in their commercial activity, which brought them great material wealth.

In England this was reflected in the flourishing of the arts, as in Shakespeare's theater, as well as science, in Newton, and in medicine, in Harvey. In the Netherlands, painters like Rembrandt and scientists like Leewenhoek emerged.

Johannes Kepler (A New Astronomy)

Kepler was born in 1571 in Weil, a small town in southwest Germany. Coming from a poor family, at the age of 15 he was fortunate to receive a scholarship from the Duke of Wuerttemberg which allowed him to graduate in Astronomy at the University of Tubingen, whose supervisor, Michael Maestlin, was in favor of the Copernican system.

In 1558 he became a bachelor and, three years later, he received a master's degree in Philosophy.

In 1594 he started teaching Astronomy and Mathematics in Gratz, Austria. Two years later, at the age of 25, he published the book *Mysterium Cosmographicum*, where he was the first to recognize that forces between bodies were caused not by their relative positions, but by their mechanical interactions.

Tycho Brahe, another notable astronomer of the time, after reading his book, invited him to work with him at the Benatek observatory, near Prague.

Eighteen months after arriving in Benatek, Tycho Brahe passed away and Kepler was appointed as his successor.

After carefully reading the movements of the planet Mars, left to him by Tycho Brahe, he realizes that the planets do not always move at the same speed, moving faster when they are closer to the Sun and more slowly when they are away from it.

In 1609, he presents his two main planetary laws in *New Astronomy*, and the third law, ten years later, in the book *Harmonice Mundi*:

1. The planets revolve around the sun, not in a circle, but in elliptical orbits, one of the foci of the ellipse occupied by the sun.
2. The planet does not move, in its orbit, at a uniform speed, but in such a way that a line drawn from the planet to the sun always covers equal areas at equal times.

3. The squares of the periods of revolution of any two planets are among themselves like the cubes of their average distances to the sun.

In 1621 he published the book *Epítome Astronomie Copernicanae* in which he presents the main results of his studies and where he states that an astronomical theory should be based on physical principles to explain the movement of the planets.

According to Koestler[49], the discovery of Kepler's laws represents a milestone in the history of science. Kepler realized that each planet was subject to two conflicting influences: the force of the sun and another force located on the planet itself. It was these two forces that now impelled him to approach the sun, now to move away from it. Today we know that these two forces are gravity and inertia, and although Kepler never formulated these concepts, he paved the way for the development of physics.

Kepler died on November 19, 1630, due to a fever where the treatment employed - repeated bleeding - only worsened the infection, culminating in his early death.

Before he died he composed the following epitaph to be placed in his grave:

The heavens I measured, and now I measure the shadows,

My soul to heaven has always been trapped,

And now stuck to the ground lies my body.

Newtonian mechanics

Isaac Newton was born in Woolsthorpe, England, on December 25, 1642, the son of a small farmer who died a few months before his son was born.

In 1646 his mother, Hannah, remarried and Newton then moved in with his maternal grandmother.

In 1653, when his mother became a widow for the second time, Newton went to Grantham school, where he learned Latin, which came to be useful in his career as a scientist.

After graduating from high school in 1661, he went to Trinity College, Cambridge.

In 1665 he obtained a bachelor's degree in Humanities, having been self-taught in mathematics because this subject was not part of his college curriculum.

At the same time that Newton was interested in science, he also cultivated a mystical side, devoting much of his time to studies on alchemy and theology.

His studies on mechanics began in the same year as his course, that is, in 1665.

Soon he realizes that to describe mechanical phenomena in a mathematical way the knowledge of the time, such as algebra and geometry, were no longer enough. It would be necessary to consider very small units of time and movement, that is, an infinitesimal amount , that is, the infinitesimal calculation . Only after the introduction of this new mathematical tool was it possible for Newton to arrive at his great discoveries.

Eurico de Aguiar

His main work, *Philosophiae Naturalis Principia Mathematica*, where his main discoveries and principles are presented, was published for the first time in 1687. It presents the foundations of the basic principles of movement and its application to planets, comets, the moon and its effects on the tides.

Newton's laws:

1st. Every body remains in a state of rest, or of uniform motion in a straight line, unless it is compelled to change that state by forces applied to it.

2nd. The change in movement is proportional to the printed driving force, and occurs in the direction of the straight line on which the force is printed.

3rd. For each action there is always an equal and opposite reaction, that is, the reciprocal actions of two bodies, one on the other, are always the same and directed to opposing parties.

Among other applications, Newton deduced that the movement of a planet is the result of competition between the tendency of the planet to move in a straight line with constant speed - if no force acts on it - and the movement corresponding to the gravitational force directed towards the Sun.

His discoveries were fundamental to the development of science in general and Physics in particular.

Since 1703, Newton has chaired the most important scientific society of his time, the Royal Society.

He was made a knight in 1703 and died on March 20, 1727, being buried in Westminster Abbey.

William Harvey (The discovery of blood circulation)

With Harvey, medicine begins a new phase. Instead of the emphasis on anatomical studies, the priority becomes physiology. Born in England, at Folkestone, on April 2, 1578, he was the eldest of eight brothers. He was the only one to pursue a medical career. He studied in Padua, where he graduated in 1602.

Fabrizio's disciple, published, in 1628, his great work: *An anatomical dissertation on the movement of the heart and blood in animals*. It deciphers the phenomenon of blood circulation.

It suggests that the heart is like a pulsating pump, which works like any muscle, contracting and relaxing. That contraction of the left ventricle causes the expansion of the aortic artery, which carries blood to the organs. That blood returns to the heart through the veins. From there it goes to the right atrium, from there to the right ventricle, which then contracts and takes blood to the lungs through the pulmonary artery. Then, oxygenated, the blood flows through the pulmonary veins to the left atrium. From there to the left ventricle, and so on continuously, without ceasing.

Another great merit of Harvey was to develop simple experiments to confirm his hypotheses. He said that the blood transported through the aorta could only come from the veins. If an animal's artery is cut, it will bleed to death. The bleeding becomes slower and slower until it runs out, and the animal dies. "The reason for death must be because the lost blood does not reach the veins, and so it cannot return to the arteries", concluded the scientist.

To explain the connection between arteries and veins, he imagined the existence of small communicating vessels between them. As in his work he never used the microscope - which was only developed at the end of the 17th century - he could not confirm the presence of blood capillaries, which was only done with the studies of Marcello Malpighi, in 1661.

He returned to England and was still recognized for his work, having been a physician to two English kings.

With Harvey, the idea arises that each organ has a function to be discovered in terms of its way of acting and its relations with other organs and the body as a whole. He died in 1657, in London, at the age of 79.

Two logical and fundamental conclusions were reached with Harvey's discovery:

- The possibility of injecting drugs intravenously.

- The possibility of replacing blood, through venous transfusion.

The first societies and scientific journals

In London, in 1662, some more enlightened English subjects decided to organize the first scientific society[50], which was sponsored by King Charles II, was called the *Royal Society for Improving Natural Knowledge*, and its founders were influenced by the works of Francis Bacon. In one of his books, the philosopher reported how a research institution should operate[51].

In March 1665, the Royal Society launched the first edition of its magazine, called *Philosophical Transactions*, which actually succeeded the *Journal des Savants*, published in Paris in January 1665. However, while *Philosophical Transactions* was interested by scientific studies, the French periodical focused on topics related to the humanities area.

Leewenhoek (The rise of the microscope)

The son of a brewer in the Dutch city of Delft, Anton van Leewenhoek was orphaned by a father at the age of 16. This forced him to take a job in a fabric factory, as an assistant accountant. It was there that he met the magnifying glasses used to count the thread threads, and which had little capacity to increase.

He only knew the Dutch language because he was unable to develop better training, due to the financial difficulties he faced.

Encouraged by his work, he began to develop magnifying glasses with increasing magnifications, polishing biconvex lenses and assembling them between two pieces of metal.

Throughout its long existence (1632 to 1723) it developed about 400 instruments, which got to produce increases of up to 275 times. With his magnifying glasses, he visualized, for the first time, the fascinating microscopic world. He examined various types of water: rain, snow, wells, rivers and the sea. From each preparation, which he kept assembled indefinitely, he tried to write down his own observations.

Regnier de Graaf, a famous doctor and anatomist of whom he became a friend, put him in contact with the Royal Society, London. Since then, Leeuwenhoek wrote hundreds of letters to that scientific society, and in 1676 he described, for the first time, the different ways in which bacteria present themselves.

In addition to seeing the bacteria for the first time, he realized that vinegar eliminated them. Today we know that the fact that there is acetic acid in vinegar is what makes it bactericidal. He also found that heat was able to kill *animacles* (a term he used for microbes).

If these two of your observations had deserved more attention at the time, certainly the implantation of aseptic surgery and antisepsis would have been implanted earlier, which only happened in the late 19th century.

The first statistics

From the 17th century, two Englishmen, William Petty and John Graunt, realized the importance of a quantitative study of health problems as a subsidy for improving the quality of life of citizens.

In 1662, Graunt published a book entitled *Natural and Political Observations Made Upon Bills of Mortality* . Their studies were based on the annual London records, which had been collected by the government and summarize these records as numerical tables for the interval between 1604 and 1661, including the presentation of the first "life table", that is, a systematic organization of data on Londoners' life expectancy.

Graunt, together with his friend Petty, created a new way of obtaining information about the population through the analysis of official data such as birth and mortality records.

Despite recognizing the precariousness and imperfection of the data he obtained, Graunt believed that if they were interpreted correctly, they could provide useful information for the development of measures that would contribute to reducing the population's mortality.

In addition, by saving lives, England would be preserving part of the considerable investment made by society in the development of people until maturity, generating, as a consequence, a greater return than any other type of investment.

Petty, a doctor in the British army who invaded Ireland in 1650, realized that the control of communicable diseases and lower infant mortality could contribute to the increase in population and that for this to be possible there would still be a need and a considerable improvement in training. of doctors. In 1676, at a conference in Dublin, he stressed the obligation of the State to promote the progress of medicine in order to contribute to improving the living conditions of the population.

In France, the mortality of children up to one year old was quite high. At the *Hospital for Abandoned Children in Paris*, between 1771 and 1777, between 31,951 births there were

25,476 deaths in this age group or an 80% mortality.

The following table refers to the births and deaths of the English city of York, England, from 1770 to 1776:

Year	Births M	Births W	Deaths Men	Deaths Women	Total
1770	237	467	203	214	417
1771	225	451	225	260	485
1772	238	490	220	288	508
1773	244	474	241	258	499
1774	214	453	173	209	382
1775	255	490	237	251	488
1776	255	498	177	219	396
T:	1668	1655	1476	1699	3175

       In this period, mortality due to problems related to pregnancy and childbirth was considerable, which, in a way, explains the greater number of deaths among women.

Art and Cure

Thomas Sydenham (The English Hippocrates)

While the trend of medicine in the seventeenth century was directed towards the exact sciences, such as physics, chemistry and mathematics, Sydenham advocated the return of the doctor to learning at the bedside of the patient.

During his existence (1624 to 1,689), many believed that the physician's main task was to devote himself to anatomical studies or mathematical calculations. Sydenham devoted his life to clinical practice.

It presented a clearer concept of the diseases, separating the main symptoms from the secondary ones. According to what he said, when a certain disease attacks the organism, it in turn tries to resist through its own defenses, the symptoms being the result of this struggle between the organism and the disease. The pain, the fever, the weakness would not be the disease, but simply the proof of the struggle and the effort that the organism makes to defend itself.

He said that every disease belonged to a certain and well-defined modality, which could be described and classified, just as a botanist does with his plants.

He described several types of diseases, such as malaria, scarlet fever, measles, pneumonia, dysentery, cholera and hysteria.

However, his main work, published in 1683, deals with gout,

a disease that afflicted him for most of his life. As a result, he wrote:

"The doctor needs to keep in mind that he himself is subject to the same laws of mortality and illness that others are subjected to; and so he will care for the sick with more tenderness, as long as he remembers that he, in person, is their companion of suffering[52]".

He was one of the pioneers in the use of cinchona bark (quinine) for the treatment of malaria, recently brought from the Inca territory, in Peru.

The fact of coming to know a medicine with specific action for a disease caused a strong emotion in the medical environment at the time. It was deduced, then, that the basic condition for the institution of an effective treatment would be a correct prior diagnosis.

Its efficiency could not be explained by any theory previously formulated, and generally mistaken, such as humoral theory, or even by the expulsion of some type of demon or haunt from the patient's body.

Like Hippocrates and unlike his contemporaries, Sydenham described superstition and mythology, insisting that the disease consisted of a natural phenomenon and as such should be resolved.

<u>Boerhaave (The Dutch Hippocrates)</u>

Hermann Boerhaave completed a medical course at the University of Leiden, and in 1701 was one of his professors, at the age of 33.

Sydenham's admirer emphasized the importance of bedside learning and a return to the study of Hippocratic texts.

In addition to teaching medicine, he was also a professor of botany and chemistry in his country.

Its most important contribution to medical knowledge was the concept of disease as a process of functional change, and not as something independent of the organism.

He realized the importance of anatomopathological studies, or that the changes that occurred after death should be correlated with the symptoms and diseases presented by the patients who are still alive.

Throughout his life he had enormous professional recognition, accumulating great fortune, in addition to leaving followers who contributed to the development of medical knowledge.

Albrecht von Haller, his most brilliant student, developed studies in several areas, was a person of great erudition, and had in the area of the physiology of blood vessels and the nervous system his greatest scientific discoveries.

John Hunter (A new surgery)

Considered, together with Paré and Lister, as one of the greatest surgeons of all time, John Hunter made the surgery move from a strictly technical level to that of an experimental science. Hunter was said to be the same for surgeons as Mozart for musicians. Before him, surgeons were undervalued by society.

Brother of anatomist William Hunter with whom he learned a lot during his life, John was the founder of pathological anatomy in England.

He introduced artificial feeding, through a flexible tube passed to the stomach, and also a device to reinforce breathing.

It innovated in aneurysm surgery, demonstrating that only by ligating the artery in the area prior to the injury would the patient be cured. Before this modification proposed by Hunter, the aneurysm was ligated at both ends and then removed, which considerably increased the surgical risk and its postoperative complications.

He published several books, including one on dentistry, in 1771, only being preceded in this science by the Frenchman Pierre Fauchard, who published his work in 1728.

In order to assess whether gonorrhea and syphilis had the same cause, Hunter self-inoculated himself with gonorrhea patient material. Unfortunately, the patient had both diseases, which contributed to maintaining the belief that they had the same etiology.

He died in 1793, after suffering a heart attack triggered by a violent discussion about the appointment of his successor at S. George Hospital.

Morgagni (The founder of Pathological Anatomy)

Giovanni Batista Morgagni (1682-1771), at twenty-nine, was a professor of medicine at the University of Padua. He published several books, the most important of which is the connection he made for the first time in the history of medicine, between the changes found in Organs diseased organs and the clinical manifestations of the respective pathologies.

He noted the anatomical differences between the normal organ and the patient, and demonstrated that, for each anatomical abnormality, a functional change corresponded.

He said that necropsies would only be useful when those who performed them had a thorough knowledge of normal anatomy and a detailed and accurate clinical history of the patient.

For him, the important thing was to look for the origin of the disease from the visible changes it would have caused in the body.

The art of healing in Brazil (The early days)

The Jesuits[53] arrived in Brazil in 1549, together with the governor-general Tomé de Souza, remaining in the country until 1759 when they were expelled by Sebastião José de Carvalho e Melo, count of Oeiras and marquis de Pombal, powerful minister of D. José I.

During the period they were here, the Jesuits were important not only in catechizing the Indians, but also in education and assistance to the sick, acting mainly as nurses and apothecaries, but also as doctors.

During catechesis, they carried out an intense campaign to discredit the shamans, until they replaced them, along with the Indians, as curators. The remnants of indigenous medical art, fused with what remains of African art, persisted only among the healers and pais-de-santo of candomblés and centers of low spiritualism.

According to Botelho and Costa[54] , "the obstacles between colonial actors, in particular, the missionaries and the shaman, the character of multiple representations and functions[55] in the intra and extra-tribal balance, they transcended the dogmatic issue that involved Christian conceptions of health and disease, because they directly interfered with the colonial project involving indigenous groups that offered greater resistance ", and the shaman's leadership among the indigenous peoples has always been quite significant.

In 1487 the Holy Inquisition was established in Castile, Spain. As a result, Portugal received, in a short time, hundreds of thousands of Jews trying to escape religious persecution. Of these, around thirty thousand were converted to Catholicism. It was the New Christians, who fled in search of a place where they could work and live in peace with their families. They managed to live peacefully in Portugal until, in 1496, D. Manuel I ordered his summary expulsion from the Portuguese lands.

Many sought exile and others remained in exchange for their possessions. In 1506, at the inspiration of two friars, there was a great killing of Jews in Lisbon, which became known as the "killing of S. Domingos", where two thousand people were murdered.

From 1531 the Holy Office was installed in Portugal, and with that several converts emigrated to Brazil, but even here they were not always able to escape religious fanaticism.

The first doctor to practice his profession in Brazil was a new Christian, Jorge Valadare s, who arrived here with the governor-general, Tomé de Sousa, as well as the apothecary Diogo de Castro.

In a letter dated 1550, Father Manuel da Nóbrega thus addressed Father Simão Rodrigues, then in Lisbon: "This land is very healthy to live; and I confirm it now, saying that it seems to me the best I can find, since since we have been here I have not heard that any died of fever, but only of old age and many of gallic illness or hydrops".

In this blessed land there were, at the beginning, two types of professionals: physicists, who practiced medicine, and barber surgeons.

In addition to the most common operative acts at the time (amputating, reducing dislocations and treating wounds and fractures), they still bleed, applied leeches, pulled teeth and also cut their clients' hair and beards. They started out as apprentices or helpers to older professionals and, after being experienced in the art, were examined. Those who were approved received the "letter from the barber-surgeon", which regulated their profession.

Physicists already studied in European medical schools, such as Coimbra and Salamanca.

There were also graduate surgeons - trained in other European schools, such as Montpellier, France -, who came here, especially in the 18th century.

The first hospital was built in Olinda, in 1540, the Santa Casa de Misericórdia. Three years later, Santos was built. Salvador's was founded in 1550. f

In the sixteenth century, there were several epidemics in our territory, with smallpox alone, which occurred in 1563, 30,000 people died in three months.

The victims of the Holy Inquisition were deported from Brazil to the Lisbon prisons, their property confiscated, tortured and encouraged to report other people, relatives or not, who later came to have the same fate as the whistleblower. Some were even denounced for the simple envy that their professional success aroused in less capable people.

The persecution would only end in 1810, after the signing of *the Trade and Navigation and Friendship and Alliance Treaty between Portugal and England*. In its article 9, it stipulated that the Inquisition would no longer reach the southern domains of the Crown of Portugal.

With religious freedom there has been a considerable improvement in the quality of life in Brazil. The emigrants started to prosper, built their cemeteries and houses of prayer.

The indiscriminate use of bleeds in Brazil only

stopped occurring after the yellow fever epidemic in 1850. So many patients died after bleeding that doctors had no more doubts about considering this practice as harmful to their patients.

The first medical books published in Brazil

Three books deserve to be highlighted as the first ones published in our country, at the end of the 17th century and the beginning of the 18th century. They are: Simão Pinheiro Morão's *Single Bladder and Measles Treaty*, published in 1683, which deals mainly with smallpox epidemics; the *Single Treaty of the Pestilential Constitution of Pernambuco*, by João Ferreira Rosa, published in 1694, which deals with epidemics of yellow fever; and the *News of what is the animal's sting*, by Miguel Dias Pimenta, published in 1707, and which deals with "mal do culo" or "mal de Angola". It describes a dysenteric disease that led to death, with gangrene of the rectum and that also used to cause rectal prolapse. Today we could speculate that these were cases of bacillary dysentery, a disease caused by bacteria of the genus Shigella, or even amoebic dysentery.

All three authors were doctors of Portuguese origin.

The historical importance of the first two books lies mainly in the fact that they are considered the pioneers in dealing with the epidemiology of diseases found in Brazil.

Eurico de Aguiar

Bernardino Ramazzini (Father of Occupational Health)

      Bernardino was born in Carpi, at the Duchy of Modena, on November 5, 1633. As a child he was educated by the Jesuits and graduated in medicine at the University of Parma in 1659.Then he practiced medicine in Modena, when he became interested in diseases associated with various types of work activities.

Although he was not the first to write a text on the health of workers, Ramazzini was the first to delve into the topic.

In 1700, he published the book *Discourse on the diseases of artisans*, where he addressed the health risks of forty-two groups of workers, from miners to surgeons. He described the links that existed between illnesses and occupations, and what should be done to reduce occupational illnesses.

There are chapters on diseases of apothecaries, bakers, millers, painters and soap makers, in addition to addressing metal poisoning that occurred with metallurgical workers and the presence of silicosis among those who worked with stones.

In the tenth chapter of his book he presents a picturesque story of sulfur mine workers. In it, he describes a case of a woman whose husband unexpectedly comes home, causing her to hide her lover under the bed and cover him with a blanket that had been cleaned with sulfur. However, the lover is quickly discovered due to the coughing and sneezing that the material residues cause.

He recommended that, in every consultation, doctors should ask patients about their professional occupations, and that this could be relevant for the elaboration of a correct clinical history.

He died in 1714, aged 81, in full professional activity, due to a stroke.

In addition to the merit of dedicating his life to the study of occupational health, Ramazzini was also an excellent clinician. He recognized the importance of parsimonious use of medicines, and said: "In inappropriate combinations there is a change in the quality of the drugs and that is why one should not combine different medicines where their compatibility is not perfectly known".

This is a valid rule until today, since the drug interaction between incompatible drugs can aggravate, instead of curing diseases.

The French Revolution

The revolution that changed the history of mankind in the late eighteenth century had among its main enlightenment mentors like Locke, with his liberal political theory; Voltaire, who was also a supporter of the liberal theory, was against any kind of religion for the wealthy classes, but not for the poor population, according to him, unworthy to be clarified. [56]; Montesquieu, with his famous theory of the separation of powers (legislative, executive and judicial), who said that virtue was the basis of democracy; and Rousseau, who, with his democratic theory, exposed in *The Social Contract*, brought the necessary legitimacy to the development of representative forms of government, as we know them today. It was also important for untying the ethics of knowledge, introducing ethical rationalism, instead of purely theoretical rationalism, as was the rule until then.

Rousseau also said[57]: "as long as only power is on one side and knowledge and understanding alone on the other, the scholar will rarely study big questions, princes will even more rarely do great actions, and the people will remain stingy, corrupt and miserable".

The French Revolution also contributed to the evolution of medicine by criticizing the method hitherto used in universities, essentially supported by the authority of books, in favor of direct observation of patients or in the emphasis on clinical examination, in the creation of hospitals and in the examination necrological[58].

The release of the mentally ill

From the French Revolution onwards, new ideas of freedom, equality and fraternity became a constant concern for most of the intellectual elite of the time.

The state of confinement and cruelty in which the mentally ill lived until the 18th century was unimaginable. They were locked up in prisons, correctional facilities and nursing homes, and watched over by ignorant people who believed insanity was the product of sin and the devil, or other causes as absurd as these.

According to Foucault[59]:

"Strange surface, which contained the measures of internment. Venereal, wanton, dissipating, homosexuals, blasphemers, alchemists, libertines: an entire nuanced population finds itself suddenly, in the second half of the 17th century, rejected beyond a dividing line, and imprisoned in asylums that will become, in one or two centuries, the closed fields of madness".

Also according to Foucault, people were even publicly whipped by people with madness, in addition to being chased in a simulated race and driven from the city with blows.

The treatment given to the mentally ill was a consequence of the ignorance, superstition and moral condemnation that surrounded him.

In 1791, Joseph Daquin published the book *Philosophie de la folie*, where he recommended the abolition of chains and confinements for the mentally ill, in addition to considering these procedures as very harmful to patients.

In Italy, Vicenzo Chiarugi published, in 1793, a book on madness, *Della pazzia in genere e in especie*, where he reports on the modifications he developed in Florence.

With humanizing treatment, with more freedom for patients, and restricted only to the most violent, it has made great progress. According to Chiarugi, mental illnesses could be divided into three groups:

Insanity, with changes in sensory activity, oscillating between melancholy, mania and dementia.

Mania, which manifested itself through the excess of audacity of the will.

Dementia or general insanity, without emotional manifestations, characterized by deficiency in both intelligence and will.

He also emphasized the importance of psychotherapy and a treatment that could both stimulate and sedate, depending on the condition of the patient, whether he was hyperactive or atonic.

However, the great reformer of the treatment of the alienated was Philippe Pinel, a doctor at the Bicêtre Hospital de Paris, who, after the loss of a friend affected by a mental illness, began to dedicate his life to psychiatry.

Convinced that a more humane treatment could be more effective, he freed 53 patients who were hospitalized with the diagnosis of insanity, after convincing the National Assembly that, in doing so, he would be in line with the ideals of the French Revolution.

In 1801 he published a medical-philosophical treatise on mental illness, where he stated that the origin of the disease was due to pathological changes in the brain. One of the most important effects of the reform of the treatment of these patients was the establishment of hospices, from the beginning of the 19th century.

Jenner (The first vaccine)

The variolization technique, which consisted of inoculating

material from a smallpox lesion in another person, with the benign form of the disease, has been known since ancient times in China. It was forgotten for a long time, until two doctors trained in Padua, Emmanuele Timoni and Jacob Pylarini, rescued her during her passage through Constantinople, Turkey, in the early 18th century.

However, it was only in 1719, through the wife of the English ambassador to Turkey, Lady Wortley Montagu, that this technique was more widely disseminated in England. She popularized variolization by publicly defending its use, including vaccinating her two children in this way. She was a very beautiful woman, until she contracted smallpox in 1717, in Constantinople, and her face was disfigured by several scars as a result of the disease.

Although it was a breakthrough, variolization was not a completely risk-free technique. Severe forms of the disease sometimes occurred after inoculation of the material. Consequently, there was a need to look for another way to make people immune to smallpox.

Edward Jenner was born in Berkeley on May 17, 1749, and was the eighth son of a pastor in the Anglican church.

Jenner was a Scottish doctor who had been interested in the study of natural history, having obtained a scholarship from the Royal Society, to study the mammal hedgehog and the cuckoo bird. In her pilgrimages to the countryside, throughout her research, Jenner came into contact with several peasant women who had acquired the bovine form of smallpox, but none of them would have acquired human smallpox. This information was essential for the development of his work.

In 1788 there was an epidemic close to the city where Jenner lived, and he then noted that people who had had cowpox also did not acquire the human form of the disease.

He continued to observe the relationship between one disease and another for 25 years, until he became convinced that he could try to standardize a protection technique against human smallpox using material obtained from the lesions of bovine smallpox.

On May 14, 1796, Jenner vaccinated an eight-year-old boy, James Phipps, with the secretion of a peasant woman, Sarah Nelmes, whose hand injuries were in the active stage of cowpox. The experiment took place as Jenner expected: six weeks after the vaccine, the boy received considerable doses of human smallpox material in both arms and still did not develop the disease.

In 1798 he published his studies on the smallpox vaccine, which were enthusiastically received throughout Europe.

Jenner demonstrated that one disease could prevent another, but it was not yet known how it happened. It was, in fact, a cross reaction between antibodies produced against cowpox, and which also managed to neutralize human smallpox viruses, due to the similarities between the two types of viruses, in terms of molecular constitution, because they belong to the same family as poxviruses. This information only became known in the second half of the 20th century.

The beginning of medical geography

Interest in the relationship between geography and health dates back to antiquity. The book of Hippocrates *on Airs, Waters and Places*, which deals with the occurrence of different diseases in different parts of the world, influenced many professionals in different periods of history.

In 1792, the German Leonhard Ldwig Finke published the work *Versuch einer allgemeinen mediicinish-praktishen Geographie (An essay on Medical-Practical Geography)*, in which he raises a series of questions little or not yet explored.

As a physician who had to visit his patients in towns and villages in his district as a duty, Finke examined water sources, surveyed sanitary conditions, produced reports on the health of the population and collected data on climate, plants and citizens' way of life.

Finke's book had three volumes, the last of which contained a manual on how to make works similar to his. Finke divides his work into a geography of diseases, a geography of nutrition and a geography of medical care.

Finke suggested that not only the geographical location, but also the size of each area should be described. Then there should be a historical section containing enough information to understand the current conditions.

Animals and plants should be determined. The region's economic, social and political structure, as well as statistical data on births and deaths, should be included. The diseases that caused the deaths should be listed, as well as the years where epidemics would have occurred.

The most frequent diseases should be described, as well as possible factors associated with them, such as climate, population habits and other information considered relevant for understanding the situation.

He said that the survey should be concluded with the presentation of government measures to be implemented to control epidemic diseases, as well as the help to be offered to the most needy population.

Hospitals should be included, if any.

Finke's work must be understood as constituting a first stage in the formation of social medicine, that is, state medicine.

Johann Peter Frank (The medical police)

Johann Peter Frank (1745-1821) published in 1778 a work in nine volumes on the Medical Police - *System der volltändigen medicinischen Polizey* - , where he made extensive use of statistics to establish the importance of the measures to be taken in public health, which he considered a duty of the State. His proposals proved to be quite influenced by the Enlightenment.

He said that misery was the mother of diseases, suggesting that there was greater concern with the assistance to pregnant women and children, care with food, clothing, housing, paving, limunination, water supply , destination of garbage and sewage, greater cleaning cities and even on the disposal of corpses . He criticized the neglect with which monarchs maintained the majority of their people.

From Frank, a new health awareness was created in several countries, leading to greater control and inspection of measures related to hygiene and health of the population.

The industrial revolution and health reform

The transition, in England, from an essentially agrarian economy to one based on industrialization[60], between the end of the 17th century and the beginning of the 18th century, it was called Industrial Revolution.

Because it was the first modern industrial country, public health reforms were also initiated in England.

Since the sixteenth century, there had been some concern among English government officials about the problem of poverty among their population. With the creation of the "Law of the Poor", the administration of each locality was responsible for supporting its destitute.

This assistance vision clashed with the liberal ideas, advocated by Adam Smith. The English theorist was the author of *The Wealth of Nations - Investigation of its nature and its causes*, a book published in 1776 that inspired David Ricardo to describe, for the first time, the concept of economic model as a simplifying abstraction of economic reality.

In his book, Smith seeks to demonstrate his belief in the growth of labor productivity, which would stem from changes in the division and specialization of the work process, providing, on the other hand, an increase in the surplus over wages and thereby allowing the accumulation of capital, a determinant variable in the supply of productive employment.

In turn, the pressure for demand for labor on the labor market, caused by the process of capital accumulation, would cause a concomitant growth in wages and, due to improvements in the living conditions of workers, there would also be improvements for the rest of the population.

The parallel increase in employment, wages and population would expand markets, which would represent capital as the basic foundation for the development of the economy.

Smith therefore believed that the market itself would regulate society and that private initiative was the source of peoples' progress.

In view of this, the assistance policy went into decline, since poverty was seen more as a consequence of the moral deficiency of individuals. For this reasoning, any aid would stimulate the leisure and irresponsibility of the poorest.

Another considerable influence for a negative view of the poor came from Calvinism, which, according to Weber[61], had a strong influence on the most developed countries in Europe in the 16th and 17th centuries. By the doctrine of predestination, the foundation of Puritan morality, divine providence would work only for those who are predestined to eternal life. And yet, according to Calvin, only as long as the people were kept poor would they remain obedient to God.

With increasing industrialization and a greater increase in the supply of jobs in cities, urban centers have undergone rapid and significant changes. Between 1801 and 1841 the population of London went from 958 thousand to almost two million inhabitants and the same happened in other English cities, like Birmingham, Liverpool and Manchester.

According to Braudel[62], "a dark England is progressing, settling in, with its feverish cities and workers' houses. Of course it is not a happy England. (...) These are huge cities, unfinished, that are being built quickly and badly, with no previous plan, but alive; this rosary of great urban centers, compact, shaking, Leeds, Sheffield, Birmingham, Manchester, Liverpool, is the soul of the English advance. If Birmingham has a human aspect, Manchester is hell. From 1760 to 1830, its population multiplied by ten, from 17 thousand to 180 thousand inhabitants. Lacking a place, the factories on the hills have five, six and even 12 floors. There are palaces and workers' houses planted at random throughout the city. Puddles of water and mud everywhere; for each paved street, ten filthy alleys. Men, women and children huddle in sordid houses; in the basements, up to 15 or 16 people live ".

Alongside this growth, the situation of urban sanitation and housing was extremely precarious. In the homes of the poor, there were often no toilets. Waste was transported in urinals to the street, where it was emptied.

In Manchester there were fifteen hundred cellars, where five people often slept in the same bed.

Low wages prevented the working class from having better living conditions. Dirt, disease, unhealthy working conditions[63] and housing, everything contributed to make life almost unbearable.

As a result, several epidemics (cholera, typhoid, typhus) emerged, which mainly affected the families of the poor.

It was also noticed that these epidemics caused a considerable economic loss, which was harmful to all and their cost represented, in fact, a waste for the State.

In 1842 a report was released whose author, lawyer Edwin Chadwick, is considered one of the pioneers of public health. It analyzed the precarious health conditions of the working population of Great Britain.

The report demonstrated a direct relationship between the poor living conditions of the poor (unhealthy housing, unclean environment, lack of drinking water and sewage supply, lack of regular garbage collection, malnutrition) and diseases that afflicted them.

It also demonstrated that a good part of these diseases would be preventable, and that the most important preventive measures to be taken related more to civil engineering and to the increase in the purchasing power of the masses than to medicine.

Chadwick's report promoted a series of positive consequences in the area of hygiene, concluding by leading to the creation, in 1848, of the General Health Council, which started to supervise and improve the sanitary conditions of each location.

In the same year, the function of public health doctor was created, the first being assigned to work in London.

After appearing in Great Britain, health reform in a short time influenced the policy of other countries in Europe and the United States of America, with public health being considered a duty of the State.

In our country, this vision only became a reality with the 1988 Constitution, as determined by art. 196: "Health is the right of all and the duty of the state".

Laënnec (The creator of the stethoscope)

René Théophile Hyacinthe Laënnec is considered the creator of the clinical diagnosis of chest diseases. His discovery of mediated auscultation was made through the use of a paper cylinder, the precursor to the current stethoscope, a word from the Greek (stethos / scopein) which means examining the chest.

As he verified that he obtained greater discernment of the sounds emitted from the chest using this device, soon afterwards he started to use hollow wooden tubes.

Two years after his discovery, he published a book on the auscultation clinic for pulmonary and cardiac diseases, in 1819. It presents, in detail, the different signs, in different diseases, obtained by percussion and auscultation.

In his book, *Treated Mediated Auscultation*, he presented excellent descriptions of tuberculosis, pneumonia, bronchiectasis, pneumothorax, emphysema, lung cancer, in addition to the sounds emitted by the heart.

He died at the age of 45, a victim of tuberculosis, a disease he described so brilliantly in his books.

Semmelweis (A martyr for hospital infection)

Ignaz Philipp Semmelweis was born in Hungary, and in 1846 he became an assistant at the First Obstetric Clinic in Vienna.

This infirmary had acquired a bad reputation, due to the high mortality rates among the puerperal women.

When Semmelweis took over the position of assistant, 36 patients died out of 208 patients, a mortality rate of more than 17%. The parturients admitted to this hospital were poor women. The rich had their children in their own homes.

The other obstetric clinic, the Second Clinic, at the same hospital, was attended only by midwives, who were trained there by more experienced ones. At the First Clinic, medical students and their professors, also doctors, worked.

In the Second Clinic, of midwives, mortality was less than 1%, according to a survey by Semmelweis.

These figures startled the Hungarian doctor, who started looking for the reason for so much discrepancy, since what was expected would be a lower rate at the clinic where the doctors worked.

On February 13, 1843, the American physician Oliver Wendell Holmes made a statement to the *Boston Society for Medical Improvement*, where he spoke about the contagion of puerperal infection, and stated that pregnant women should never be seen by doctors who had performed necropsies or attended to cases of puerperal infection.

And yet, that the disease would be transmitted from one patient to another. In addition, it would be efficient preventive measures for medical assistants to wash their hands with calcium chloride solution, and change their clothes after attending to a case of puerperal infection.

This communication by Holmes provoked violent opposition from local doctors, who did not accept it.

Despite not being aware of Holmes' work, Semmelweis continued to try to discover the cause of his paradox.

In 1847, his pathological friend, Kolletschka, died days after being injured during an autopsy, after cutting his finger with his scalpel.

Upon reading the description of the necropsy of his friend's body, he found that the picture was identical to that of patients who died of puerperal infection.

He concluded, then, that the high mortality rates should be caused by something that the students would bring from the autopsy room, contaminating the hospitalized women. As in the Second Clinic, midwives who did not attend the pathology room would not bring this contamination, which would explain the differences in mortality found. At this time, the theory of germs causing infectious diseases was not yet known.

As a result, from May 15, 1847, Semmelweis began to demand greater rigor in the attitude of infection prevention. He placed a sign at the entrance to the First Clinic saying that every doctor or student, without exception, was obliged to wash their hands with chloric acid solution before entering the obstetric clinic, when coming from the necropsy room.

Despite many complaints and widespread misunderstanding, Semmelweis managed to get his orders carried out, and in a few months the rates dropped to 3%.

Later, he found that in addition to the transmission of the disease occurring from the dead to the living, it could also happen among living patients, through the hands of doctors. It inaugurated a new phase of its struggle, determining the most rigorous disinfection of the hands, after each exam.

He supervised the sterilization of the instruments, which until then had been cleaned in the surgeons' overcoats, in all hospitals at the time, and started to remove the parturients with inflammatory processes in isolation units.

In 1848, the mortality rate of the First Clinic decreased, for the first time, to 1.33%.

Despite the success achieved, Semmelweis acquired many enemies with his crusade. With that, he had to leave Vienna that same year and went to Budapest, his hometown.

In 1860 he published his findings on puerperal fever in a book that was badly received by doctors. Only one or the other voice rose in support. Five years after publication, he began to show signs of mental insanity, suggestive of schizophrenia.

He died in 1865, victim of septicemia, after injuring his finger in his last autopsy, similarly to what happened to his friend Kolletshcka.

The emergence of Homeopathy

Until the end of the 18th century, the therapeutic arsenal of medicine was very limited. Quinine was used against any type of fever, as well as mercury chloride (calomel), which was even used to treat syphilis.

Art and Cure

In addition, patients had to undergo heroic procedures, based on bleeds (leeches, suckers or even venipuncture), purgatives and emetics, in addition to vesicles, where irritating substances were placed on the patient's skin, causing burns and then infections. It was believed that, in doing so, doctors would be eliminating the impurities responsible for diseases.

During this period, many patients died more from the consequences of the aggressions suffered with the treatments than from the diseases themselves.

George Washington, President of the United States of America, received on December 17, 1779 the following treatment for a throat infection: in the morning, he suffered a half-liter bleed, without showing improvement; soon another doctor was called, applied vesiculation on the neck and removed another half liter, also without result; two other doctors came and made another bleed, of a liter, in addition to administering mercury chloride. At 10 pm, the illustrious patient passed away.

It was in this scenario that the German doctor Samuel Hahnemann appeared. In 1790, he laid the foundations of homeopathy, after translating the book *Matéria Médica,* by William Cullen, a professor at the University of Edinburgh, Scotland.

Unlike Cullen, who believed that the effect of quinine (from which quinine was extracted) was due to an action in the stomach, Hahnemann would have been surprised to try the drug on himself and find that its effects were similar to those that appeared on his own disease she cured.

From there, he launched the principle that the similar is cured by the similar, and that the more diluted - or dynamized - the more active the medicine is.

With these two basic foundations, Hahnemann's method was extraordinarily successful, since its therapy was not iatrogenic as the rule of medicine used then. In 1823, he was forced to leave Leipzig, due to the hostility of the city's apothecaries and doctors, who felt hurt by him.

It was in this historical context that homeopathy emerged. It was clearly superior to allopathy because it did not aggravate the patient's condition. However, with the development of chemotherapy, homeopathy was losing ground to allopathic medicines, which made homeopathic medical schools almost disappear after the first decades of the 20th century.

According to Hahnemann's theory, the therapeutic effect of its formulations could not be gauged by the physicochemical properties of the drugs, since they depend on the concentration of the molecules of each substance.

However, the attempt to explain it through the argument that dilutions - dynamizations - would release an "internal energy" from the remedies does not find a scientific basis capable of supporting it.

Other authors try to explain the action of these drugs, stating that they would mobilize alternative reserves of the organism itself. It is difficult to understand which reserves would be regimented differently by homeopathic and allopathic medicines. Immunity does not seem to be capable of making such subtle discrimination.

According to the poet Heine, homeopathy is useful in the diseases of love, where one must apply the principle that the like heals the like, or a new love is the best remedy for a failed love.

The beginning of homeopathy in Brazil

In 1840, Dr. Pedro Chernovitz, a Polish doctor who emigrated to Brazil, expressed himself about the situation of doctors in Rio de Janeiro: "If I start to think about my profession, I see how the people are mistaken, thinking that the wind of good fortune lifted me above the crowd. But most are hardly able to earn a living. There are, therefore, many who would not be able to survive if they had no other income".

It was in this context that homeopathy appeared in our country. In December 1843, the Frenchman Benoit Mure, trained in medicine at Montpellier and who later studied with Hahnemann himself, founded, in the capital of the Empire, the Homeopathic Institute of Brazil.

Due to the difficulties experienced by doctors here, it was to be expected that there would be a strong reaction against the new way of treating diseases.

Homeopathy was not only more accessible to the poorest strata, which homeopaths often attended free of charge, but also a welcome alternative to the aggressive methods of official therapy.

Benoit Mure soon became the target of the demoralization campaigns of those who believed they were harmed by the emergence of this new professional competition.

He was accused of having bought his diploma and even of murdering his stepdaughter. He was also denounced for illegal practice of medicine, patient poisoning and other minor slander.

With this, their attempts to legalize the teaching of homeopathy were blocked in parliament.

In addition to the struggle for a disputed labor market, the corporate struggle of doctors was also due to divergences in content that have always placed allopathic medicine and homeopathy in opposing fields throughout history.

Mesmer and animal magnetism

Through treatment with the imam, Franz Anton Mesmer developed a form of treatment that was widely accepted in the 19th century. His method, also called mesmerism, was nothing more than a type of suggestion, hypnosis or "nervous sleep" [64].

His tendency towards the unusual could be seen in the thesis with which he concluded his medical course: The *influence of stars on human bodies*.

The principle, according to Mesmer, was based on a force that emanated from the doctor, that existed in all living beings and that allowed to establish mutual relations between them. With the help of this force, one organism could modify another through the action of the will.

Because of its exteriorization, comparable to the strength of the magnet, he called it "animal magnetism". Rubbing magnets on patients' limbs, he believed to provide an influence similar to that exerted by the gravitational action of the Earth.

In the works of Isaac Newton, published previously, the physicist said that there is "a subtle spirit that permeates and lies at the core of all dense bodies; due to their strength and performance, the physical particles attract each other". Probably these works influenced the doctor a lot.

Through the application of the hands, or by hand passes, Mesmer intended to cure nervous disorders directly, and indirectly all others.

Some of his followers made a fusion between mesmerism and religion. According to this type of association, the patients who could be cured by magnetism would be only those who were pure and free from sin. And also, only the doctors blessed by God could use this great magnetic force.

Even today, some religions that use a pass use Mesmer's technique in order to free people from their ills, as well as from demonic possessions.

On the other hand, some claim[65], that Mesmer's contribution was relevant because he foresaw the importance that the unconscious plays in our lives. Thus, despite his eccentricities, Mesmer could be considered a precursor to Freud.

Beginning of experimental research in physiology

From the end of the seventeenth century, medicine ceased to be concerned only with the study of anatomy and began to focus also on the first studies of physiology and pathology in a more scientific way.

There were works for the detection of insensitive perspiration, done by the Italian Santorio Santorio (1561 to 1636) and later by other researchers like François de la Boe, also called Sylvius (1614 to 1672), author of interesting studies on the role of saliva, pancreatic juice and bile in digestion.

The Dutchman Cornelius Bontekoe (1614 to 1687) said that the thickening of the blood was responsible for a great number of diseases. To fine tune it, he recommended the use of tea. He was later criticized for having interests in promoting the product due to his relationships with wealthy Dutch tea traders.

Albrecht von Haller (1708-1777), from Berne, carried out several works on the physiology of muscular activity. He developed the concept of irritability, involving nerves and muscles.

After the discovery of oxygen, by Scheele and Priestley, after Cavendish demonstrated that air was an almost constant mixture of nitrogen (78%) and oxygen (21%), Lavoisier (1743 to 1794) proved that both combustion and breathing, imply oxygen consumption from the air, with carbon dioxide emission at the end. He also recognized that the heat produced in metabolic exchanges depends on the oxidation of carbon by the animal organism.

Most important diseases until the end of the Modern Age

Tuberculosis

Long before causing disease in humans, tuberculosis was endemic in animals since the Paleolithic period. The agent that caused infection at that time would probably be Mycobacterium bovis (M. bovis), which causes disease in cattle and which can be transmitted, through milk, to other species.

As man began to adopt agriculture as a regular mode of production - around 7,000 BC - he began to settle in clusters and to domesticate some species of animals, such as cattle, pigs and goats. Thereafter, tuberculosis emerged as a disease in humans, but still in an infrequent form.

As previously mentioned, several Egyptian mummies were found showing mycobacterial infection.

As cities grew larger, the environmental conditions for the transmission of the disease also increased, changing the weak balance that existed between the bacillus and the individual.

It is believed that the human tuberculosis bacillus, Mycobacterium tuberculosis, originated from M. bovis, as a mutant, and that it was introduced in Europe in the 16th century.

After the elimination of those most sensitive to the bacillus, through selective pressure on the human species, an increasing proportion of the population showed resistance to infection and it started to present, predominantly, an endemic picture of chronic lung disease.

The bacterium continued without causing major problems, in terms of disease, until Europe's environmental conditions, from the 17th century onwards, made it possible to spread among large urban agglomerations of people who lived in basements, with high promiscuity and little chance of spreading. protect from the cold.

These conditions have never before been found to this extent in the history of mankind.

From then on and until the end of the 18th century and the beginning of the 19th century, the epidemic grew and spread throughout Europe and North America, with deaths due to tuberculosis reaching 25% of the total, at its peak.

In South America, Asia and Africa the situation reached its climax in the early 20th century, or about a hundred years later.

Cholera

The history of the capital of England is strongly linked to the River Thames, to which it owes not only its foundation, but also a good part of its economy for being one of the centers of commerce and international communication, in addition to serving for transportation, recreation, food and water supply.

Despite the beauty of the river and the wealth it brought to the city, there were considerable difficulties in collecting water for home use and, until the 17th century, London was supplied mainly with water extracted from shallow wells that were excavated both from public places as well as private areas, such as backyards and gardens.

Then, until 1830, nine private companies were responsible for serving 164 thousand tenants, in a city with around 200 thousand houses and an estimated population of 1.5 million people, with the Thames being the source of collection for all these companies.[66].

Before the beginning of the 19th century, complaints about water quality were few, mainly because people from the upper classes, who had political strength, used private supply companies and rarely used this water to drink in its raw form., that is, in its natural state.

In their homes, water was used predominantly for washing and cooking. At the time, beers were the drinks most used by a large part of the population, including those that were made at home.

In addition, only around 1828, the conditions of the River Thames began to deteriorate considerably, and already that year there were about 140 sources of sewage directly polluting the river.

Edwin Chadwick, famous lawyer and responsible for the beginning of the English public health legislation, in his *1842 Health Report*, considered not only the conditions for collection but also the storage of water in the areas where the working classes lived.

The water supply in these areas had as main source shallow wells with valves and the water was then carried to households in buckets or vases, which were often uncovered and exposed to different environmental conditions.[67].

Chadwick's report had repercussions among some doctors, such as the surgeon Joseph Toynbee, who in 1844, before the *Royal Commission on the Health of Cities*, stated that based on his own investigations "he was convinced that the quality of the water, the mode of transmission and the atmosphere in which it was maintained influenced the health of the population to a much more serious extent than had ever been imagined before.[68]".

John Snow was born in York, England, on March 15, 1813 and was the eldest of a family of nine children of a worker and his wife, who lived in conditions considered to be modest.

At the age of 14, with the help of an uncle, he left York and went to live in Newcastle, already with the firm purpose of graduating in medicine.

In the new city he started working at the local infirmary and soon managed to become assistant to the pharmaceutical surgeon William Hardcastle, an experience that lasted for five years.

In 1831, he had his first impactful contact with a cholera epidemic, during which he treated several patients in one city, Killingsworth, whose economy was linked to coal mines.

On that occasion, he found that the disease could affect a still healthy person in the morning and that, after a day of agony, he would die at night, an experience that would forever mark his life.[69].

After completing his apprenticeship with Dr. Hardcastle in 1836, he moved to London where he enrolled at *Hunterian School of Medicine*, where he studied until the end of the course.

While still a student he wrote some scientific articles, such as one with the title "on asphyxia and the resuscitation of newborn children", in 1841.

In 1843 he received a bachelor's degree and, a year later, in 1844, he obtained his Doctor of Medicine degree from the University of London, going on to work as a surgeon and general practitioner in the Soho district.

After beginning his clinical practice, he remained interested in issues involving breathing, seeking to develop inhalation devices to be used in anesthesia.

Snow had been particularly impressed by the results obtained by William Morton, a dentist who, in 1846, with a rudimentary inhalation mask, used ether for surgeon Edward Gilbert Abbott to perform, at Massachussets General Hospital, the first anesthetic surgery in history of medicine, the extraction of a vascular tumor from the neck of a young patient.

In a short time he became a respected anesthetist, having even been responsible for the anesthesia of Queen Victoria in two of her births, using chloroform, that is, Prince Leopoldo, in 1853 and Princess Beatriz, in 1856.

But despite receiving some prestige and recognition for his work as an anesthesiologist, what continued to arouse Snow's interest were the studies on cholera.

During the fall of 1848 there was a second epidemic of the disease in England, which resulted in a considerable mortality rate.

Although, at that time, the miasma theory was still the most accepted by its contemporaries [70], Snow doubted its validity due to the fact that, through his studies, this theory was not compatible with the initial picture he found among patients with the disease.

Knowing the physical and chemical effect of gases, he believed that such a theory was at odds with a disease whose initial signs and symptoms were not linked to the respiratory tract, as would be expected by the dominant theory of its time.

On the contrary, the exuberant symptoms of cholera were focused on the gastrointestinal tract, that is, patients had abdominal pain, vomiting and diarrhea.

As a result, he correctly concluded that it should be ingested by people, which would lead them to develop the typical condition of the disease.

Based on the record of deaths that occurred in 1848 and 1849, he found that it was in the southernmost neighborhoods of London where the highest mortality rates were found, much higher than those in the rest of the city, as can be seen from the analysis of table 1 of your own work.

Table 1. Cholera deaths in London, recorded from September 23, 1848 to August 25, 1849[71]:

Sectors	Population	Cholera deaths	Rate
West	300,711	533	1.77
North	375,971	415	1.10
Central	373,605	920	2.46

East	392,444	1597	4.07
South	502,548	4001	7.96
Total	1,945,279	7466	3.84

He also noted that the inhabitants of that region obtained water to drink in a place below the River Thames, where the waters were highly contaminated by the city's sewers, a situation that differed from the other regions that received water from less contaminated sectors, in a place higher than the river or its tributaries.

With this, he established his hypothesis that cholera was transmitted by ingesting a "morbid matter" invisible to the human eye and that it should act in the intestines, producing a diarrheal condition with severe dehydration.

When drinking contaminated water taken from the river, people ingested the "morbid matter" and, as a result, became ill.

Snow published his hypothesis for explaining the disease in a short text: " *on the mode of communication of cholera* " and which, despite all the wealth of information, had little repercussion among doctors in England.

William Farr was already a respected physician in England, when in 1839, by official determination, he became responsible for investigating the causes of death and thus, more than any other, he began to develop and analyze mortality statistics in order to better outline the main health problems and most important diseases in your country[72].

In 1852, Farr published additional data on deaths in 1849, including eight possible variables with the potential to explain the causes of the epidemic among 38 districts in London.

Its variables, among others, included the number of people per acre, the annual income per household, the elevation of the residence in relation to the river level and the water supply company per household.

After studying all the possible implications of each one, he believed that the association with elevation was the most important, concluding that "the elevation of soil in London has a more constant relationship with cholera mortality than any other known element"[73].

Farr had been impressed by the fact that in the riverside districts the average mortality rate was three times higher than in the inner city districts.

This, despite having still recognized a certain association between the disease and the source of water supply in each district, although this association did not cover - in his analysis - the effects of the elevation, that is, it linked the infection inversely to the elevation in relation to the water level of the Thames.

By his analysis, the districts with the highest number of deaths were those closest to the river level and those with the least deaths were those with the highest level.

As Farr was much more respected and influential than Snow, and because his explanation did not contradict the theory prevalent at the time, that of miasmas, his theory was soon accepted by the public health system and by the vast majority of doctors as being the correct one.

However, a new epidemic of the disease, which occurred between 1853 and 1854, would forever change the way in which they differed about its causes.

Under the influence of Snow's studies, one of the companies that distributed water in the south of London, *Lambeth Water Company*, began, from 1853, to collect the product in an upstream area, where the waters were not yet polluted by the sewers of the city. City.

The other company, *Southwark and Vauxhall Water Company*, kept its collection at the same original point, that is, in a polluted area.

With this information, made available by Farr, Snow realized that he could - with the study of data on deaths by households and respective water supply companies - prove his hypothesis.

The new table 1 summarizes the data from his investigation and which were published, in the second edition of his book, in 1855:

Table 1. Rate of cholera deaths, per household, in relation to water supply companies in the southern region, compared to those in the rest of London:

Water supply company	Households	Cholera deaths	Deaths per 10,000 households
Southwark and Vauxhall	40,046	1,263	315
Lamberth	26,107	98	37
Rest of London	256,423	1,422	59

In this way, Snow proved that the deaths that occurred in households in the southern region and that received water from the company that collected it in polluted areas of the river, *Southwark and Vauxhall*, were more than eight times greater than those of the households that received the product in areas not yet contaminated by London sewers, that is, the water collected by *Lamberth*.

Another episode that also contributed to making Snow's hypothesis more accepted was the issue of the *Broad Street* water pump.

In September 1854, in a sector of London called *Golden Square*, there was an epidemic outbreak of cholera of great intensity that caused the death of 500 people in just ten days.

Connoisseur of the area, Snow knew that most of its inhabitants received water from a public pump located on *Broad Street*.

Consistent with his hypothesis, Snow imagined that the epidemic outbreak should be due to the ingestion, by the local population, of contaminated water from this pump and decided to investigate what could have happened.

Another fact that caught his attention was the information, made by popular people, that the day before the water supplied by the pump had a bad smell.

Initially, he registered the names and addresses of 83 people who died of cholera, based on death certificates and visited some of the homes, asking their residents where the water they had drunk came from.

He soon found that most of these residents were supplied with water from the *Broad Street* pump.

It also calculated the distance between the home of each deceased person and the nearest bomb, verifying that *Broad Street* was the closest in 73 of the cases, and that 61 among the 83 people who died drank from their contaminated water steadily or occasional, that is, the vast majority of deaths would be related to that bomb.

Quite satisfied with the findings of his investigation, Snow soon afterwards presented his findings to the local health authority, who immediately banned the *Broad Street* fountain by removing its water pumping lever.

Snow knew that this measure, despite generating immediate protests from the popular, would serve, if the incidence of the disease decreased, to prove his theory.

To illustrate his investigations, he also made a map of the deaths and their respective addresses, graphically demonstrating the spatial relationship between cholera deaths and the suspected bomb of contamination.

Subsequently, a local study showed that 20 feet below, that is, just over 60 centimeters from the ground, a sewer pipe passed a short distance from the pump's water source, with infiltrations on both sides of the water courses.

As a result, the complaint of a bad smell from the water coming from the pump was also explained.

After the interruption of the collection of contaminated water, there was a reduction in the incidence and mortality due to the disease, but popular pressures and the lack of support from the health authorities - still adherents of the miasma theory - made the *Broad Street* bomb return soon after. used to the general detriment of the local population.

Only after Snow's death did his theory come to be partially accepted, when Farr published his monograph on the epidemic that hit London in 1866.

In it, it attributes the spread of the disease in four ways: through personal contact, through air, through vapors emitted by sewers and water[74].

Despite remaining, in a way, still partially faithful to the miasmatic theory, as when he attributes some responsibility to the air and sewage gases, Farr, for his respectability, contributed in a fundamental way to make Snow's theory more welcome by the community scientific and health authorities of the time.

Thus, we can conclude that the discovery of cholera transmission resulted from the convergence of Snow and Farr's works, that is, despite the fact that from the beginning Snow had the correct theory, it can only be confirmed with the support of the obtained statistical data. by the health surveillance system developed by Farr[75].

The modern art of cure

There is no people without history or that can be understood without it.

Eric Hobsbawn

Nineteenth century philosophical ideas

Some philosophers were more influential on the development of society, and especially of science in the 19th century: Kant, Hegel, Comte, Marx and Nietzsche.

Imannuel Kant (1724 to 1804), one of the most important modern philosophers, had as a principle that each man should be considered as an end in itself, a way of presenting the doctrine of human rights.

He is considered the founder of criticism, a method of philosophizing that consists of investigating the sources of his own statements and objections and the reasons on which they are based. Kant said[76] that "the first step in the things of pure reason, that which characterizes your childhood, is dogmatic. The second step is skeptical and helps to circumspect judgment, driven by experience. But a third step is needed, that of mature and manly judgment".

Kant was an ardent defender of freedom, and said that "there can be nothing worse than one man being subject to the will of another".

In his most important book, *The Critique of Pure Reason* (1781), he seeks to prove that, although nothing of our knowledge can transcend experience, there is still a part of understanding that does not depend on the senses. It is the ability to form, create or perfect knowledge due to the nature and structure of pure reason, which exists a priori. This knowledge covers not only logic and mathematics, but still much that cannot be included in it, nor deduced from it. In the same book, Kant defined the synthesis as "the act of joining different representations to one another and conceiving their multiplicity in the form of a unique knowledge".

Towards the end of his life he published the book *A Perpetual Peace,* where he advocates the creation of a federation of free states, to sign an agreement to end the war. According to Kant, war could only be prevented by installing an international government.

Georg Wilhelm Friedrich Hegel (1770-1831) claimed that nothing is completely real, except the whole. Nothing can be entirely true unless it concerns reality as a whole.

The whole is called by Hegel *The Absolute* and it is spiritual. *The Absolute* is not static, but dynamic, and develops according to its fundamental internal law: dialectics.

In the text *Phenomenology of the Spirit*, he formulates his conception of the process of formation of consciousness as a result of the interaction of three basic elements, which later came to influence other philosophers:

1. Moral relationships, that is, the family and social life.
2. The language, or the symbolization processes.
3. Work, or the way man relates to nature to extract his means of subsistence.

Hegel's work is so relevant that it influenced both right-wing sectors - such as when it supports conservative policies - as well as the left - when it serves as an inspiration for philosophers like Feuerbach and Marx - or in the use of dialectics to understand reality and build knowledge.

Dialectical movement is one that is made according to a thesis (affirmation), an antithesis (a negation) and a synthesis. It is through the dialectic movement that the world moves forward. Hegelian dialectics considers synthesis as a step towards overcoming the contradiction between thesis and antithesis.

According to Hegel, the reason is the conscious certainty of being the whole reality. In his separation a person is not entirely real, but what is real in him is his participation in reality as a whole. As we become more rational, this participation increases.

For Hegel, the most important was the state. He would be the embodiment of rational freedom. He also said that the whole spiritual reality, possessed by each citizen, would only be made possible through the State.

History has great relevance for the German philosopher, the way of understanding the subject being an essentially historical process. Thus, each conscience is an awareness of its time, having also been the first to elaborate a philosophy of history.

Auguste Comte (1798-1857), French philosopher, created the positivist system, which was a kind of anti-metaphysical revolt, or metaphysical skepticism. We should limit ourselves to the positively given, to the immediate facts of the experience, running away from all metaphysical speculation. There would be only one knowledge and one knowledge, which would be that of the sciences. Only science could penetrate the aspects of the world accessible to experience. Thus, philosophy would be no different from science. It would only be the coordinator of the results of the different types of sciences, seeking their harmonization. According to Comte, there were only three methods of philosophizing: the theological, the metaphysical and the positive. The first would be the starting point of human intelligence, the third, its perfect state, and the second would serve only as a transition stage.

Regarding the relationship between philosophy and science, it can be said that "science removes the difficult essence of the facts underlying the problems of the world and life, and enlightened philosophy provides the necessary safeguards to dispel illusions"[77].

Marx, like Comte, regarded metaphysics in a derogatory way, and said that "philosophers have so far done nothing but interpret the world in different ways; now it is a question of transforming it ". There are those who consider this claim by Marx the turning point in the history of political theory, when philosophy became ideology. He believed that the transformation of societies takes place through its own internal contradictions, its analysis based on two methodological bases, historical materialism and dialectical materialism.

For Marx, history must be analyzed based on infrastructure (material, economic resources, etc.) and class struggle. Consequently, it does not accept the interpretation that history is made by the isolated action of certain people, but through the conflict of interests considered antagonistic, such as those of feudal lord and servant or capitalist and proletarian.

In his main work of economics, *O Capital*, whose volume I was published in 1867, he argues that labor is the true source of all value and that profit results from the exploitation of the worker through the "extraction of surplus value", or that is, of the value created by the worker beyond what is necessary to pay him a mere subsistence wage, as was the reality of capitalism throughout the 19th century.

Nietzche, considered "the philosopher of relativism", established the intellectual bases of existentialism and a radical historicism that characterizes the modern age.

Strongly influenced by Schopenhauer, at the age of 24 he became professor of philology at the University of Basel. The main targets of its attacks were God, morality and democracy.

In the book *Ecce Homo*, he calls himself "the first immoralist". In another book, *Genealogia da Moral*, published in 1887, disputes the basis of Christian morality, such as the notions of good and evil.

It describes the altruistic virtues of the Christian tradition - such as piety, self-sacrifice and personal sacrifice - in a derogatory way, or just as a reaction of those inferior to their condition. The values that Jews and Christians defend are, according to him, "a morality of slaves". He also regrets that this morality has prevailed over time over the "morality of masters", that is, that of the ancient Greek warriors, who believed to be contained in the desire for power and in their continued search.

Louis Pasteur and the germ theory

"The creative scientist has a lot in common with the artist and the poet. Logical thinking and analytical skills are necessary attributes for a scientist, but they are far from sufficient for creative work. Those intuitions in science that led to great technological advances were, of course, not derived from pre-existing knowledge: the creative processes on which science progress is based operate at the level of the subconscious". This statement by physicist and biologist Leo Szilard[78] can perfectly adapt to Pasteur, who was undoubtedly one of humanity's greatest geniuses. Born in the French city of Dôle, he was the son of a craftsman who had been a sergeant in Napoleon's army.

Patriot, he invested his energies and, for this reason, contributed significantly to solve practical problems of various industries and agriculture in France.

With a brilliant scientific intuition, he developed research in several areas. He graduated in chemistry and, at the age of 26, established the existence of molecular asymmetry in acid crystals, such as tartaric acid.

In 1856, due to problems in the French beverage production industries, he was called in to try to resolve an issue that was causing them great damage. From time to time, wine or beer soured.

Using his microscope, Pasteur observed that, when the fermentation of sugars proceeded normally, producing alcohol, there were rounded shapes. When wine went sour and lactic acid was produced, long bacilli appeared.

He also discovered that the spherical shapes were fungi (yeasts), responsible for the production of alcohol. With the result of his research, fermentation proved to be the result of the action of living microorganisms and not a purely chemical event, as was believed until then.

He demonstrated that by heating the wine for a short period, at a temperature between 55 and 60ºC, the inconvenient bacilli died without, however, changing the properties of the wine. Pasteurization was discovered, a disinfection principle still used today for the treatment of milk.

In 1857 he realized that certain microorganisms did not grow in the presence of air, but only in their absence (anaerobic), while others multiplied only when there was oxygen (aerobic). His publication, which received the title *Mémoire sur la fermentation appelée lactique,* can be considered one of the hallmarks of microbiology.

This discovery by Pasteur was extremely important for medicine, as it led to the conclusion that putrefaction was a consequence of the activity of microbes, similar to what occurred in fermentation. Thereafter, some surgeons began to use procedures aimed at preventing postoperative infections.

Continuing his work, Pasteur demonstrated the existence of microbes in the air. And that these could contaminate liquids or solids causing their deterioration. If, however, the air were filtered, or even if microorganisms were eliminated, as through boiling, without allowing new exposure to air, nothing happened and no germs were observed.

At the suggestion of chemist Antoine Jêrome Balard, of whom he was an assistant, Pasteur used flasks with a "neck of a swan neck" in his experiments, which allowed the heated air to escape, without, however, allowing the entry of new bacteria and fungi. This was fundamental to definitively refute the theory contrary to yours.

With this, Pasteur demonstrated that the theory of spontaneous generation had no basis, despite being accepted by scientific society since Aristotle.

Between 1865 and 1868 it helped the French silk industry to eliminate two diseases, *pébrine* and *flacherie*, which were causing great losses. It demonstrated the microbiological character of the two and how to avoid them.

One of Pasteur's great discoveries was to have realized that, through successive passages in laboratory animals, or even only in culture media with variation of the optimal incubation conditions, it could increase or decrease the capacity of microorganisms to cause diseases.

Knowing this principle, he used it to produce vaccines against bird cholera, the anthrax bacillus and against the rabies agent. He never got to know the microorganism responsible for this disease (the rabies virus can only be seen by electron microscopy), despite having managed to develop a method capable of preventing it.

On July 6, 1885, he applied the rabies vaccine for the first time to an eight-year-old boy, Joseph Meister, bitten fourteen times by a dog with hydrophobia, two days earlier.

The boy's parents asked Pasteur to save his son. He then gave the boy 12 injections of the vaccine, with increasing potency, gradually, over two weeks.

The boy survived, despite the scientist's fears. A few weeks later, he presented his report on rabies prevention at the Paris Academy of Sciences. In one year the vaccine was applied to 350 people who had been bitten, with no deaths.

Pasteur's fame soon spread to the international community and his method was recognized as a major medical breakthrough.

From then on, he received the support of all French and world society for the whole of his work, of such significance for humanity.

He received donations from several countries, which allowed him to create the Pasteur Institute in Paris, from where several generations of great scientists emerged, who, like him, contributed a lot to the progress of science.

Pasteur died in 1895, and the admiration he receives from the French, to this day, is unparalleled by any other character in the history of France.

In 1940, the same Joseph Meister, who had been vaccinated when he was eight years old, was the curator of the Pasteur Institute in Paris.

When the Germans, during World War II, demanded the keys to the mausoleum built in honor of the founder of the Institute, Meister committed suicide by not accepting that someone would violate the grave of the great hero of his homeland and to whom he owed his own life.

Charles Darwin and the theory of evolution

Son of englishmen, Charles Robert Darwin was born in Shrewsbury, England, on February 12, 1809. At the age of eight he lost his mother. His father, who was a doctor, as well as his paternal grandfather, convinced him to study medicine at the University of Edinburgh, but what really delighted him was the study of plants and animals. He left medical school because he did not see anything in this career that interested him.

He graduated in Arts in January 1831, at Cambridge. The reading of Humboldt's voluminous text (*Personal Narrative*, with seven volumes and 3754 pages), in which he recounts his trip to South America, made a strong impression on Darwin. From then on, he started wanting to travel all over the planet, especially in regions that are still little explored, where, according to Humboldt, "there should be new species of plants and animals still unknown".

In 1831, at the age of 22, he was chosen to be the naturalist of the ship Beagle, who would spend five years traveling around the world. It was a small vessel, 27 meters long, 7.5 meters wide, with ten bronze cannons and 73 crew members.

The main continent studied was South America, mainly the Galapagos archipelago, close to the coast of Ecuador.

He was in Brazil, during the year 1832, having visited Salvador and Rio de Janeiro. Wherever he went, he described species, observed nature, relief and climate. He wrote down everything he found.

After five years of traveling, and several notebooks, he spent some time reflecting on the material he had collected. It was the doctrine of the population of Malthus[79] - *Essays on population* - extended to the world of plants and animals, which leads to the conclusion of his research that resulted in the book *The Origin of Species*, published in 1859.

In his book, Malthus says that all species of animals produce far more offspring than can survive. But that more offspring is necessary, because there is a lot of waste. Life is difficult and only a few remain.

The theory of Darwin is based fundamentally on the evidence that in the battle for life only the best adapted survive, which led him to develop the theory of natural selection. And, furthermore, that the environment is the main stimulus for natural selection, that is, overpopulation and competition (for food, sexual partner, group leadership, etc.) would lead to natural selection, where the most well adapted to the environment would emerge as the victors of the "war of nature". Or to summarize, we could say that only the most capable members of each species survive the gradually changing elements of the environment. They adapt to change, while the weakest - or least able - do not.

He dismissed the earlier idea that species were fixed, and that animals and plants were originally created as we find them today.

The application of his theory put an end to the anthropocentric theory, that the universe was created for man. It represented for the 19th century the same as Galileo for the 17th century.

Darwin found that nature lives in continuous transformation, that species evolve and that the emergence of new species results from descent with modifications.

In this way, the survival or not of the offspring would depend on the characteristics of the environment, and this would be the importance of natural selection. Only those with new characters would remain, while those that did not have them would be extinct.

He also believed that there was a significant participation of sexual selection, which would also contribute for the best adapted to survive.

Although he initially did not consider the contribution of Jean Baptiste Lamarck, who preceded him in evolutionary theory, important or that the different forms of life had gradually developed, starting from a common origin, in the later editions of his great book Darwin did his due recognition to that scientist.

Lamarck wrongly believed that the variations produced by the effects of the use and disuse of certain organs (the function makes the organ) in response to external stimuli (first law), and by the direct inheritance of these changes (second law), would contribute to heredity acquired characters and, consequently, for the selection of the most qualified.

The classic example of the law of use and disuse is "the neck of giraffes that grew so that they could feed on the leaves of the tall trees in the region in which they lived".

In part , because there was still no knowledge of genetics in its day, Darwin's theory did not contemplate the possibilities that mutations could add to natural selection. And yet, that many characteristics of animal and plant species would not necessarily have any value for their survival, but their work had profound significance in several areas of knowledge, and especially for the biological sciences.

Among the consequences of the theory of evolution for the development of biology can be mentioned research to try to find new drugs against multiresistant bacteria, or the genetic improvement of grains to find seedlings that are more resistant to pests.

We now know, through molecular genetic studies, that we are more like chimpanzees (the difference between the two types of DNA is less than 1%) than we imagined. Meanwhile, the difference between chimpanzee and gorilla DNA is 3%, or about three times greater. It is possible that humans and chimpanzees had a common ancestor about five million years ago[80].

Claude Bernard (A great physiologist and biochemist)

Claude Bernard was born in 1813, in France, in the village of Saint Julien. His father produced homemade wines, but ended up going bankrupt and having many debts. So at the age of 16, Claude Bernard got a job in Lion.

His boss, Mr. Millet, was a pharmacist and one of the drugs he prepared was called terga. This mixture of several and surprising components (sometimes even with more than one hundred substances), was used as if it were a panacea, which made the young employee doubt the art of healing of his time.

At the age of 19, he decided to change his life and, demonstrating literary pretensions, he embarked for Paris carrying in his suitcase a play in five acts.

There, he looks for a famous critic, Mr. Saint Marc Girardin, to whom he hands the manuscript. To his surprise, he says the following: "My dear, literature is not a trade with which to earn bread. I can say that I was more successful than many people, but if I could go back, I would enroll in medical school. Do what I should have done, sir".

Claude Bernard took the advice of the literary critic and soon after started to study medicine. After graduation he started to work at the Hôtel-Dieu, in Paris, with François Magendie, one of the great physiologists of the time. He did not, however, have the talent and brilliance of his disciple, who overcame the master with numerous works of enormous importance for the health sciences.

Bernard developed a series of researches, especially in the area of metabolism and physiology. He described the importance of liver glycogen in regulating blood glucose. Glycogen is a reserve of glucose in the body. Whenever the blood sugar level decreases, the liver releases glucose into the circulation from glycogen.

He also did work on the sympathetic nervous system (responsible, among other things, for increasing our heart beats), described the importance of pancreas secretion in the digestion of food (fats, sugars and proteins) and developed studies in the fields of pharmacology and toxicology.

However, the main biological concept that Claude Bernard developed was to describe the organism's tendency to maintain the balance of the internal environment, even if the external conditions are adverse. Our glands, through their hormones, work towards this balance, homeostasis.

Claude Bernard died in 1878, after having dedicated forty years of his life to laboratory research. His discoveries went beyond his own time.

The death of pain

Before the discovery of inhaled anesthetics, surgeons used alcohol, hashish or even opium intoxication, taken by mouth, exceptionally, in cases where complete muscle relaxation was required.

The norm, however, was surgery without any type of anesthesia. Some still tried hypnotism or mesmerism (or suggestion).

There are reports of emergency surgery, such as amputations of a limb as a result of an open fracture, in which physical methods were used, such as placing the limb on ice or even producing ischemia, with the use of a tourniquet.

There were also cases in which the production of unconsciousness was caused by a blow to the head or by means of strangulation, which attenuated the production of pain even at a high cost to the patient.

However, the method most used to achieve a relatively smooth surgical field was, simply, restraining the patient by force. It does not take much imagination to realize that surgery was seen, then, as the last resort in treating patients.

In the United States of America, Crawford W. Long persuaded a young man, James M. Venable, to inhale sulfuric ether while removing a small tumor from his neck - an infected sebaceous cyst - on March 30, 1842. The surgery had three witnesses: Andrew Thurmond, William Thurmond and Edmund Rawls.

His knowledge of the effects of the drug came from his student days, through demonstrations made by Chemistry teachers with their own students.

Long continued to use ether in several other surgeries, but the scientific community knew nothing about the episode, until the fact was reported in an article published in 1849 in the *Southern Medical and Surgical Journal*, where Long claimed to have applied ether to some patients in his office, in the small town of Jefferson, Atlanta, during 1842.

Nitrous oxide was synthesized by Priestley in 1776, but despite its anesthetic properties since 1796, it had never been used in surgery. Its use was restricted to the production of euphoria, like a perfume launcher that was used in the carnivals of old.

While watching a kind of circus show where people inhaled nitrous oxide to make them laugh, on December 10, 1844, dentist Horace Wells realized that one of those who had inhaled the gas had seriously injured his leg, without, however, manifest having felt any kind of pain.

He quickly came to the conclusion of the meaning of this finding. The next day, Wells, who besides being a dentist was a medical student, had one of his own teeth extracted, by an assistant, without pain. Whoever applied the anesthesia with nitrous oxide was responsible for the show, Gardner Colton.

From there, Wells began to spread the good news around the world. However, in one of his demonstrations of the anesthetic power of the gas, it failed, probably because the anesthesia induction time was too short, or because the anesthetic dose was small.

One of his students, William T. Morton, who witnessed the master's failed attempt, learned from Charles Jackson, an internationally known physician and chemist, the anesthetic power of sulfuric ether. After experimenting with it on animals, on September 30, 1846, in his office in the city of Boston, he did a dental extraction on one of his clients, without pain.

Soon the fact was widely publicized and, on October 16, 1846, Morton anesthetized, using a kind of rudimentary inhalation mask, Edward Gilbert Abbott, while John Collins Warren, a famous surgeon at Massachusetts General Hospital, performed the extraction of a vascular tumor of the patient's neck.

At the end of the surgery, without the patient having expressed any pain, Warren said to the students who had seen the operation: "Gentlemen, this is not a scam".

On November 16, 1846, the feat was announced in an article published in the *Boston Medical and Surgical Journal*.

Morton tried to patent the use of ether as an anesthetic, but ended up failing to do so.

After the introduction of ether, new experiments followed using chloroform, mainly in the obstetric clinic. The first person to use this anesthetic in obstetrics was the Scottish physician James Young Simpson, who was also the pioneer in the use of ether to relieve labor pain, in an experience that took place on January 19, 1847, in a patient who was suffering violent pain. , during a very complicated delivery.

Later it was found that chloroform is toxic to the liver and produces severe cardiovascular depression. Its only advantage over ether is that it is not flammable. Even so, it was used a lot, for almost a hundred years, mainly in Great Britain.

The effect of the discovery of anesthetics was fundamental for the development of surgical specialties. Before, the surgeon had to be extremely fast, in addition to rarely the patient being relaxed and without showing great suffering, which made it very difficult to develop the skills of the surgeons.

The lives involved in discovering the surgical use of anesthetics have not had a happy outcome.

Wells became addicted to chloroform and committed suicide in 1848, in Tombs prison. Charles Jackson died at the age of 75, in 1880, in a Sommerville hospice, where he lived for seven years. Long was not recognized for the primacy of using anesthesia in surgery and died impoverished after the American civil war. Morton died in 1868 of a heart attack, poor and bitter because he was unable to patent the use of ether or the device he had invented for inhaling the anesthetic.

A monument erected by the citizens of Boston on Morton's grave, in a cemetery near the city, has the following words on its headstone:

Inventor and disseminator of inhalation anesthesia

Eurico de Aguiar

Before him, at all times, surgery was agony

Through it the pain in surgery was avoided and canceled

Since then science has started to control pain

Rudolph Virchow (And cell pathology)

He graduated in medicine in Berlin in 1843, Virchow founded the magazine *Air quivos of Pathology,* in 1847.

In his first work published in this journal, he said that an unproven hypothesis of any kind represented the same as a boat too fragile to sail and dismissed the notion that any man was infallible about judgment or knowledge.

A person of great culture and varied interests, Virchow worked in areas as diverse as anatomy, pathology, epidemiology, public health, anthropology, archeology, teaching and politics.

In 1849, when investigating a typhus epidemic in the interior of Germany, he was very impressed with what he saw. Then he published an indignant account of the miserable conditions in which the workers lived. This cost him his job, but it did not dampen his fighting ability.

In this report, he attributed the cause of the epidemic to social deprivation, poverty, illiteracy and social and political inequality. In his opinion, only through democracy, education and social justice could these other similar epidemics be better controlled.

For his liberal positions he was elected parliamentary, next to the Reichstag, in the period from 1890 to 1893.

In medicine he developed the theory of cell pathology - "every cell comes from another cell" - which said that the disease site should be looked for in the cell, whereas the macroscopic and microscopic changes in the organism were a consequence of the cells' reaction to the causes of each disease.

Each part of the sick body maintained a parasitic relationship with the rest of the healthy body to which it belongs, and which would live at the expense of the organism. This concept is correct, especially in chronic degenerative diseases, such as cancer.

The doctrine of cell pathology, first described in 1858, was based on the study of living structures and the observation that the microscopic appearance of living cells changed profoundly with the disease.

If we assume that healthy life is due to the normal functioning of cells, including their metabolism, it is reasonable to believe that changes in the functioning and shape of these cells cause the body to become ill. In this case, the organism would become ill from a subclinical stage (where signs and symptoms of the disease would not yet appear) to the clinical stage (where there would already be clinical manifestations of the disease).

On his 80th birthday, Virchow received an award of 80,000 marks, in addition to a gold medal offered by the Emperor of Germany, in recognition of his great contribution to the development of science.

He died in 1902, when the largest hospital in Berlin was named after him.

Robert Koch (Founder of Bacteriology)

One of the thirteen children of a German mining supervisor, Koch was born in 1843, and graduated in medicine in Göttingen, having been a student of Jacob Henle, considered one of those responsible for the development of the contagion theory.[81]. He served as a medical officer during the Franco-Prussian war. Then, in 1872, he went to a small town, Wollstein, close to the Polish border.

There, isolated from the scientific community, and working in an improvised laboratory, separated from the office by a curtain, Koch developed a series of research that revolutionized bacteriology and, as a result, medicine.

His microscope was a birthday gift from his wife. He developed a primitive method of making good quality microphotographs and improvised an incubator.

In his day, the culture media used in bacteriology were liquid, which made bacterial isolation extremely difficult.

To make it feasible to work with only one type of bacteria at a time, Koch decided to add gelatin to the medium and, with that, began to improve his technique. Then he started using agar, which allowed the culture media to solidify at room temperature, without compromising the viability of the microorganisms he worked with.

With this big step, Koch began to isolate several bacteria that cause infectious conditions. He developed studies with the anthrax bacillus, with the bacillus that causes hemolytic septicemia and, in 1878, published the results where, for the first time, he demonstrated that the cause of six different diseases in animals were six different bacteria. And that only one form of bacteria was found in each disease.

For these studies he was awarded a high rank and a laboratory in the Department of Imperial Health in Berlin, in addition to gaining the support of two assistants.

Today, it is known that while still at Wollstein, he worked on the development of the microscope, together with Ernst Abbe and Carl Zeiss, having been the first scientist to have a microscope equipped with the light condenser and the immersion lens developed by the two exceptional experts optical. This innovation was extremely important for the development of Koch's works, as they allowed the visualization of bacterial structures that no other instrument allowed at the time.

From there, his research could develop more quickly. New staining methods and new isolation techniques came to allow him to visualize the tuberculosis bacillus, for the first time in 1882, from cultures developed in the blood of sheep.

His discovery was presented in Berlin, on March 24, 1882, in a scientific meeting that perplexed the entire audience made up of Germany's most famous doctors.

In the same year, he published the results obtained in the journal of the Physiological Society of Berlin, where he also included his postulates to consider a certain agent as the cause of a given infectious disease:

1. May the microorganism always be found in the disease.
2. May the microorganism not be found in other diseases, or in health.
3. Let the microorganism be cultured artificially and reproduce the disease in question, after inoculating a pure culture of the agent in a susceptible animal.
4. That the microorganism can be recovered from the animal so inoculated.

Like Pasteur, Koch was a patriot. Several times, the two, together with their respective assistants, disputed the privilege of the discoveries of the new science they helped to create.

In the case of cholera he was the winner. In 1883, researching an epidemic in Egypt, he was the first to isolate Vibrio cholerae.

In 1888, Koch and his wife Emmy separated, due to the little attention he paid him. She remarried again in 1893, to a beautiful young 21-year-old art student, Hedwig Freiburg, with whom he fell in love when he saw her in a portrait painted by an artist.

Its greatest failure, however, occurred during the 10th International Medical Congress, in 1890, when it announced tuberculin (the current PPD) as the cure for tuberculosis. Although it is still used today as a test to assess immunity to the bacillus, tuberculin could not be considered as a therapeutic weapon, as was soon demonstrated.

In 1905 Koch received the Nobel Prize for medicine. He died in 1910 as one of the founders of bacteriology, along with Pasteur.

The consequences of advances in bacteriology, physiology and pathology

The emergence of bacteriology has led to a new era of medicine. The clinician and the surgeon were forced to make major changes in the way they think and reason about diseases, their causes, symptoms and treatment plans.

The theory of cellular pathology also contributed to the great changes that occurred in medicine during the 19th century.

They significantly influenced the concepts of etiology, nosology and immunology of diseases.

The study of the cell made us aware that it was in the sphere of the microscopic world that the solutions to the most important medical problems would be.

The new discoveries in physiology and biochemistry (in addition to other basic areas) brought the conviction that it was in the research carried out in the laboratories, and not in the clinic, that would be the basis of the progress of medicine.

With the considerable development of science, there was a tendency towards specialization, as it became increasingly difficult to retain so much, and more and more frequent, new information about so many and so varied fields of scientific knowledge.

The general practitioner, who would dominate all fields of medicine, became increasingly rare.

Gregor Johann Mendel (Founder of genetics)

The son of peasants, he was born in Austria in 1822. He graduated as a priest in 1847. Four years later, he went to the University of Vienna to study physics, mathematics and natural sciences. Back at the convent where he graduated, in Brünn, Czech Republic, he began to dedicate himself to his famous breeding experiences between different varieties of peas, through which he was able to discover the first laws of heredity.

Today it is known that the characters found in the different varieties of peas are defined by segments of deoxyribonucleic acid (DNA), and are called genes.

The gene is the hereditary unit that is transmitted to the offspring by each parent, and that will be responsible for the appearance of a certain character or characteristic in the child, along with the partner's gene.

In higher organisms, genes occur in pairs. The genes are united within a larger structure, the chromosome. There are alternatives to a gene, which are called alleles. The alleles occupy the same position on homologous chromosomes.

Mendel's Laws:

Dominance law: in hybrids, one of the opposite characters, or alleles, dominates, masking the other, which is recessive, in a certain proportion.

Law of character segregation: the opposite characteristics of the ancestors dissociate, in the following generations, according to fixed proportions, that is, 25% of pure dominants, 50% of hybrid dominants and 25% of pure recessives.

Law of the independence of the characters: in the crossing of races or varieties that differ by more than one characteristic, each characteristic is transmitted independently of the others.

Published in 1865 in the Brünn Society of Naturalists magazine, Mendel's work went unnoticed until 1900, when botanists Hugo de Vries, Carl Correns and Erik Tshermak von Seysenegg independently reached the same conclusions as he did.

Mendel died at the Brünn convent in 1884, without having received the recognition he deserved from his contemporaries.

Between 1912 and 1926, Thomas H. Morgan, from Columbia University, promoted a great development of genetics using breeding experiments with fruit flies, of the species Drosophila melanogaster.

Its life cycle is short (around twelve days) and fruitful (an average of 1,000 eggs). Flies can have white or red eyes, the white characteristic being linked to the X chromosome, and of recessive character, coming to appear mainly in males, similarly to what happens with color blindness in humans.

They have four pairs of chromosomes, including a pair of sex chromosomes. Analyzing the results of the crosses of the flies,

Morgan was able to construct a physical map of each chromosome, showing the relative location of each gene.

In 1933, Morgan came to receive the Nobel Prize in medicine, and one of his students, Muller, for mutation-inducing work in Drosophila, using X-rays, came to receive the same prize in 1946.

Currently, we know that the DNA contained in the total of 100 trillion cells in the human body, if extended from one end to the other, would be 40 times the distance from Earth to the Sun, although in each of our cells the DNA is found. if condensed into a core about 0.005 mm in diameter.

The art of healing in Brazil in the 19th century

The arrival of the Portuguese royal family to Brazil also had good consequences for the evolution of medicine. At the insistence of Dr. José Corrêa Picanço, first court surgeon, D. João VI created, in 1808, in Salvador (February 18), and later in Rio de Janeiro (April 2) the first medical and surgical academies in the country . Before, those who wanted to pursue this career had to study in Coimbra or in another European college.

Picanço, one of the two Brazilians who taught at the Faculty of Medicine of Coimbra (the other was José Francisco Leal, professor of the subject of Materia Medica e Farmácia), had the chair of anatomy under his responsibility. He later went on to become Baron of Goiana, as a prize for his contribution to the Portuguese Crown.

The course lasted five years, with anatomy, chemistry, physiology, hygiene, etiology, pathology, therapeutics, operations, obstetrics and medical clinic. At the end of the course, the student received the title of approved surgeon.

In 1832, D. Pedro II transformed the academies into medical colleges, and the course was extended to six years, with a more improved curriculum. The subjects then taught were as follows:

1) Medical physics.

2) Medical botany and some notions of zoology.

3) Medical chemistry and some notions of mineralogy.

4) General and descriptive anatomy.

5) Physiology and hygiene.

6) External pathology and external clinic.

7) Internal pathology and internal clinic.

8) Topographic anatomy, operative medicine and devices.

9) General medical material, and especially Brazilian, pharmacology and therapeutics.

10) Forensic medicine, application of medical sciences to legislation.

11) Childbirths, diseases of women and children.

12) History of medicine, methodology or exposure of different medical systems and explanation of Hippocrates' aphorisms.

The internship took place in the last two years of the course, and the history of medicine was given only during the sixth year.

At the end of the course, after defending a thesis on a clinical or surgical theme, the student received a doctor of medicine degree.

The courses were eminently theoretical, with a lack of didactic material and adequate facilities.

From the 19th century onwards, France began to have a greater influence on our sciences, as well as on literature, commerce and customs in general. This ancestry prevailed until the middle of the 20th century, when American culture began to exercise the leadership that it maintains until today.

The creation of public health laboratories in Brazil

Pasteur's example with the creation of his Institute in Paris, focused on the research of infectious and parasitic diseases, had consequences in several countries. Many researchers were trained at that center and, upon their return, created similar institutes.

In Brazil, the Bacteriological Laboratory, which would later be called Instituto Adolfo Lutz in honor of its first director, was created in São Paulo, in 1892. Lutz graduated in medicine in Bern, Switzerland, having taken training courses in several European cities. From 1889 to 1892 he was responsible for the treatment of leprosy in Hawaii.

In Rio de Janeiro, the Soroterápico Institute of Rio de Janeiro was created at the same time, with headquarters at Fazenda de Manguinhos. To direct him, the mayor appointed Baron de Pedro Afonso. Soon after taking over the direction, the baron traveled to Paris with the purpose of hiring a scientist from the Pasteur Institute to be his technical manager.

There, he was surprised to learn from Émile Roux, who succeeded Pasteur in the direction of the Institute, of the existence, in Brazil, of a researcher who fully met the conditions. Returning to Rio, the baron hired Dr. Oswaldo Cruz, who had remained from 1896 to 1899 at the Pasteur Institute, where he went to improve his knowledge, especially in bacteriology.

The Institute's headquarters was completed in 1900. In the famous Moorish-style palace, the administration of the institution is still today.

In 1902, Oswaldo Cruz assumed the general direction of the institute, which started to undergo considerable expansion, hiring a team of young researchers of great capacity, such as Carlos Chagas and Adolfo Lutz. Lutz left São Paulo in 1908 to work in Manguinhos, until he died in 1940.

In Belém, in 1936, the Northern Experimental Pathology Institute was founded. In 1940 it became known as Instituto Evandro Chagas, in honor of its director at the time, son of Carlos Chagas, who, like his illustrious father, was a great researcher of tropical diseases, having died at the age of 35, in an air crash. The Evandro Chagas Institute is today, in virology and other areas of tropical medicine, one of the main references in Latin America.

Joseph Lister (Antisepsis and asepsis in surgery)

-My husband will be so happy! Repeated Agnes Lister to the

foreign visitor several times. His colleagues are indifferent ... Everyone believes that the current conditions in hospitals come from God, or from nature, and that nothing should be changed. Others see no way but to wipe out hospitals, as if they were to blame for all the death[82].

The visitor was a German surgeon, Henrich Hartmann, who had learned of Lister's experiences in 1865, adopted shortly after he learned of Pasteur's work on putrefaction caused by anaerobic bacteria.

Joseph was the son of an English wine merchant, Joseph Jackson Lister, who used his leisure time to solve optical problems, including several improvements to achromatic lenses, lenses that transmit light without fragmenting it into its component colors, and that led to a great development of microscopes.

Lister graduated in medicine in London in 1852. In 1856 he married Agnes, the eldest daughter of Prof. James Syme, from whom he learned surgery in Edinburgh, Scotland.

At that time, it was believed that there was healthy pus after surgery. Surgeons believed that the presence of purulent secretion helped the wound to heal.

Lister, however, based on his own statistics, was impressed by the high mortality rates. In amputation surgeries, 45% of patients died, and in other types of operations the rates were also very high. Opening the chest and abdomen, then, was the same as certain death.

From then on, he started looking for ways to reduce this scourge.

In 1863, he became aware of the work of a French chemist, Jules Lemaire, who published a book on the medical value of carbolic acid (phenol) and from there he started to vaporize the operating room with this disinfectant, while using it in the field. operative and soaked it in the linen dressings he applied after surgery.

He was also extremely demanding with cleaning, from the operating rooms to the wards. With the scalpel he used to buckle (sterilization by the heat of a flame), at the suggestion of Pasteur himself. Generally, surgeons cleaned the scalpel on their apron, in addition to using the same scalpel for several patients.

What Lister did not have, like the other doctors of his time, was the knowledge that the bacteria that caused surgical infections, in most cases, were from the patients' own normal skin microbiota. The use of phenol eliminated these germs, acting as an antiseptic, and therefore infections did not develop.

Lister's results were very satisfactory, with a sharp drop in the postoperative mortality rate, and his data were published in 1867, in the Lancet magazine, with the title *On a new method of treating compound fractures, abscess, etc., with observations on the conditions of suppuration* .

In 1869 he succeeded his father-in-law as a professor of surgery in Edinburgh. In 1877, he assumed the chair of surgery at the University of London and, in 1897, he became the first doctor to have a seat in the House of Lords.

He died in 1912, and his remains are kept today in Westminster Abbey, as well as Newton.

Although at first it was widely criticized, in a few years its asepsis and antisepsis method started to be adopted by all surgeons.

As a result of Lister's work, we can mention the introduction of sterilization of surgical gowns by moist heat (autoclave), in 1886, by the German Ernst von Bergmann, and the introduction of sterile rubber gloves in 1890, by the American surgeon William Halsted.

Halsted developed the rubber gloves to protect the hands of the nurse who assisted him in the operating room, and who later became his wife. He was also the first to use cocaine as a local anesthetic, having become addicted to this drug, which ended up jeopardizing his brilliant surgeon career. In 1899 the drug was replaced by novocaine, and was no longer used for anesthetic purposes.

The beginning of scientific dentistry

In 1563, Bartolomeus Eustachius published a book with thirty chapters, containing anatomical studies of the teeth, where he stated, for the first time, that permanent teeth had their own origin, and did not have the same roots as milk teeth, as was believed time.

Ambroise Paré, the famous French military doctor of the 16th century, made an important contribution to the development of oral surgery by introducing gold or silver prostheses for the closure of palate defects.

Until the 18th century, dentistry was practiced only by surgeons-barbers, graduated surgeons and practitioners of all kinds. The professional activity was limited to the extraction of decayed teeth, almost exclusively.

From the book by the French doctor Pierre Fauchard, *The dental surgeon* , in 1728, it became clear the need for specific training for anyone wishing to work in this area.

Phillip Pfaff, a dentist for King Frederick II of Prussia, published in 1756, in Germany, another book that had a great influence on the practice of dentistry. He described how to make plaster models from wax prints. Prostheses were generally made of wood, by artisans, precursors to prosthetics.

The English surgeon John Hunter published, in 1771, another important book for the development of dentistry, *The natural history of human teeth* .

Modern dentistry emerged in the United States in the 19th century, with the first dental school in the world founded in 1839, the Baltimore College of Dental Surgery.

The introduction of anesthesia by two American dentists, Wells and Morton, contributed significantly to the progress of dentistry, as well as to surgery. In 1899 novocaine was introduced, which started to be used as a local anesthetic.

The Society of Dental Surgeons of New York, created in 1834, was the first scientific society of dentistry in the world.

In some countries like Italy, Spain and Portugal, dentistry is still a medical specialty today. To be a dentist, you must first take a medical course.

In most countries, however, dentistry is an independent science, due to its high degree of specialization and the various techniques it deals with.

Billroth and experimental surgery

Theodor Billroth developed the concept of experimental surgery, working on his new concepts first in the laboratory, only after being tested and approved to start using them in the operating room.

He was professor of surgery in Vienna, having successfully performed his first abdominal surgery on January 29, 1881, under anesthesia with chloroform. The patient, Thèrése Heller, underwent a gastrectomy due to a tumor. The operation lasted 90 minutes and the patient recovered without problems.

At that time, abdominal surgery was tantamount to a death sentence. Billroth and his team also performed 41 resections due to stomach cancer, successfully in 19 cases.

A new nursing

Until the end of the 17th century, nursing existed more as an activity linked to religious orders, and in a precarious way. Hospitals were also precarious, although there was order, discipline and some hygiene.

From that period until the middle of the 19th century, laypeople were totally unprepared, performing their functions in an amateur way. At that time, hospitals were filthy and patients died more from infections acquired there than from illnesses that led them to hospital.

It was a pastor, Theodor Fliedner, who together with his wife decided to create a nursing school in 1833, having transformed part of his residence into an asylum for liberated prisoners. In 1836 he founded the first nursing school for religious women in Germany. Florence Nightingale was one of his students.

Born in Florence, and daughter of Englishmen, she played a very important role in the development of her profession.

The Crimean war was a conflict between Russia and an alliance of England, France, Turkey and Piedmont. It was started in 1853 and lasted three years. The situation of the Allied soldiers was dire. There were many deaths, reaching more than 40% among the injured.

At the request of the English minister of war, Florence was assigned to command a body of 38 nurses in Scutari, in the Constantinople neighborhood, in 1854.

There, working in an improvised hospital - in fact an abandoned barracks where a thousand soldiers could be accommodated, but where four thousand were huddled - managed to promote major changes, which led to a considerable improvement in the survival of the wounded, with some reporting that the rate of mortality would have dropped to 2%.

As soon as he arrived, he found a place with a dirty floor, covered with dust, with windows always closed, where there was no laundry and where the doors, which closed every night, were only opened in the morning, for the removal of the dead. During the night, no one was on duty to care for the sick.

Early Florence sought to change the situation. He faced the military bureaucracy firmly and decisively and completely changed the situation he had encountered. He began to more efficiently manage the conditions of the wounded, taking care of improving the food served to them and clothing, to protect them from the cold, in addition to other basic needs of a hospital.

Florence's work was soon widely recognized and, on her return to England, she received the sum of fifty thousand pounds, which she used to found the nurse school at St. Thomas Hospital on June 15, 1860. Her students, after trained, filled all the vacancies in the great English hospitals.

Nightingale defined nursing simply as having the objective of "helping the patient to live". It also made a major contribution to the emergence of a new nurse, focused on public health.

In 1893, he drew attention to the need for health nursing and insisted that the nurse, in addition to caring for patients, should also be a health missionary, acting as a visitor and giving health guidance in homes, that is, combining the role of nursing with that of health educator and social worker.

<u>Natural medicine</u>

Natural medicine uses the diagnostic procedures of traditional medicine, but it differs from it in its interpretation of the origin of diseases and in its therapeutic approaches.

For naturalists, the disease is a curative reaction and its symptoms (fever, diarrhea, hemorrhages, etc.) are only manifestations of the body's defense.

For them, traditional therapeutic conduct is wrong because it does not correct the imbalance caused by the violation of natural laws and, on the contrary, it still aggravates the evil.

It admits the existence of diseases caused by microorganisms, but believes that they are produced after the body loses its natural balance, due to the retention of toxic products.

Among the current practices of medicine, we can mention the approach to nature, physical exercises, hydrotherapy, avoiding the ingestion of processed foods, such as sausages, the ingestion mainly of vegetable origin and not contaminated with pesticides (organic), in addition to trying to avoid overeating, alcoholic beverages and smoking.

As a result, medication intake should be viewed only as a last therapeutic resource.

In 1796, Cristoph Whilhelm Hufeland published *Macrobiotics*, which is still considered a classic of naturalism. It contains the basis of natural medicine.

Naturalism is directly related to the vegetarian regime, being based on the intake of fruits, cereals, vegetables and milk. The vegetarian doctrine has its origin in Germany, with Theodor Hahn (1824-1883), author of the books *The paradise of health* and the *Manual of healthy life.*

The rise of Pediatrics

Pediatrics emerged from the 19th century, as a branch of internal medicine. Previously, doctors treated adults and children alike. In 1850, infant mortality in France was around 20%, having remained at that level until the end of the century. Infanticide was common at that time, as was the abandonment of newborns. These children, left at the doors of the churches, invariably died. As a stopgap, "abandonment wheels" were created, installed near the doors of the convents. In 1830 there were 230 of them, and in 1833 alone, thirteen thousand children had been abandoned by this means. The last "abandonment wheel" was closed in 1868, due to the substantial fall of this deplorable practice.

The first pediatric hospital appeared in 1802, *Les Enfants Malades,* in Paris. Pediatrics has followed two parallel courses since the beginning: childcare or child growth and development and the specialty responsible for treating children's diseases. In 1815, a study based on seven thousand cases, defined the importance of knowing the child's weight at birth and that this represented a good indicator for the diagnosis of prematurity.

The first incubator was developed by Stéphane Tarnier, at the Port Royal Maternity Hospital, in 1880. Tarnier was the first to realize that the survival of premature infants required isolation, extreme hygiene, proper nutrition by nasal intubation and a humid atmosphere.

An important cause of infant mortality, which reached up to 80%, was gastroenteritis caused by contamination of bottles. With the introduction of new milk treatment techniques, such as pasteurization, infant mortality among children breastfed with bottles was equal to that of those who received breast milk.

There was also a considerable reduction in mortality from infectious diseases. In 1884, the introduction of anti-diphtheria serum caused mortality from the disease to drop from 73% to 14%.

The last enemy of surgery

The three historical enemies of the evolution of surgery were pain, infection and hemorrhage.

The first was won by the discovery of inhaled anesthetics, by Wells and Morton.

The second was partially overcome[83] by Pasteur, von Bergman and Lister, through the development of aseptic technique (use of sterile material) and the use of antiseptics in surgery.

The problem of hemorrhage still needed to be solved, which often led the patient to shock (a sharp drop in blood pressure) and then to death.

Before the evolution of hemotherapy, transfusions between different species (sheep to man) and even between those of the same species were attempted, with results, often disastrous.

In 1900, Karl Landsteiner defined the path to be followed to overcome the hemorrhage. He found that human blood is divided into four large groups (A, B, AB and O), and that transfusion accidents could be avoided if the blood of the donor and recipient were compatible, or if there were no antibodies in the circulation group against the antigen (protein that induces the formation of antibodies) of another blood group.

In 1930, Landsteiner received the Nobel Prize for Medicine for his great contribution to the treatment of anemias and hemorrhages.

In 1940, together with Wiener, Landsteiner discovered another blood group, called Rh factor (Rh positive and Rh negative), named because this factor was found primarily in Rhesus monkey red blood cells.

Another important stage in the development of hemotherapy was the discovery that the cooled blood, and containing an anticoagulant (sodium citrate), could remain viable for several weeks, which facilitated its storage and the possibility of being used at any time, even in cases of emergency.

Later, with the discovery of the leukocyte histocompatibility complex, the HLA system, by French researcher Jean Dausset, paved the way for organ transplantation, due to the reduced risk of rejection among people with similar HLA systems.

The beginning of diagnostic imaging

Wilhelm Konrad Röntgen was born in 1845, in Germany, and graduated in physics in Zurich. He was professor of the subject in several European universities.

Experimenting on the conduct of electricity in gases, he observed that, in the middle of the darkness, a paper screen covered with barium platinocyanide, close to the vacuum tube (covered with black cardboard) with which he worked, had fluorescence.

He later discovered that it was the emission of an unknown type of radiation, which was able to penetrate dense bodies, impenetrable by the waves of visible light, providing the formation of images on a fluorescent screen and a photographic film negative.

Röntgen gave the name of X-rays to this new radiation for not knowing its origin.

In fact, X-rays are electromagnetic radiation of short wavelength, which propagate in a straight line, with the speed of light, ionizing matter, including air, and can pass, be absorbed or be reflected by matter, depending on the atom used. The radiation is produced in a tube where an electric current stimulates the negative pole (cathode) to release electrons, which are attracted to the positive pole (anode), where they collide abruptly, releasing energy. Of this kinetic energy, 99% of it turns into heat and only 1% into X-rays. Without the electrical stimulus, there is no radiation emission.

Röntgen's first X-ray was taken from his wife's left hand, where the bones and the wedding ring could be seen. It was an unclear image, but the bones of the fingers were perfectly visible.

Since its beginning, radiology has made a great advance in the diagnosis of several diseases and injuries, such as pneumonia, various types of cancer and fractures.

In 1897, bismuth as a radiopaque compound was introduced in the study of the gastrointestinal tract of animals. Later it was also used in humans and, from 1904, it was replaced by barium.

In 1929, sodium iodide was first used as a contrast in arteriographies, which greatly helped in the location of tumors and other brain injuries.

Röntgen received the first Nobel Prize in Physics in 1901. He died in 1922, practically forgotten by the new generations.

Harrison (Creator of tissue culture)

Ross Granville Harrison was born in Pennsylvania on January 13, 1870. Considered brilliant by his contemporaries, he soon became interested in the study of embryology at John Hopkins University.

Then he went to Germany, where in 1899 he graduated in medicine. In 1907, working with live nerve cells, in aseptic conditions, he managed to keep them for up to four weeks. His work was published in 1907 in the *American Journal of Anatomy*, entitled *Observations on the living developing nerve fiber.*

Although he never received a Nobel Prize, Harrison's work allowed medicine to make a big leap, as when viruses were grown in cell cultures. As a result, they favored the development of several vaccines, such as those for polio, influenza and measles. His work also contributed to genetics, which still uses cell cultures to carry out chromosomal mapping.

Ehrlich (Founder of modern chemotherapy)

The son of a hostel janitor, he was born in 1854 and graduated in medicine in 1878. Early on, Paul Ehrlich became interested in chemistry, due to the influence of a relative, his mother's cousin, Carl Weigert, a pathologist who introduced the microscopic techniques of staining, with aniline derivatives.

He developed a series of researches in the most diverse areas. He had a predilection for studying dyes. He believed that if they were able to stain the microbes, they could also (when associated with molecules capable of causing damage) lead to their destruction.

In 1889 he went to work, as an assistant, with Koch. He developed a staining technique that allowed a better visualization of the tuberculosis bacillus and that was based on the alcohol-acid resistance of Mycobacterium.

Together with another German, Emil von Behring, he developed the passive production of antibodies (serotherapy) against diphtheria. As Behring patented this technique, which made him very rich, the relationship between the two became strained and distant.

He developed the so-called side chain theory, which was the precursor to the modern theory of the formation of antibodies and also served as a guide for the development of new drugs, from an original compound.

He used this strategy to look for a drug that would cure the most diverse infections and parasites.

From an organic substance, in a ring, with a side chain containing an arsenic atom (atoxil), he began to make changes in its chemical structure, aiming to discover the drug capable of eliminating all diseases.

In the version of his theory related to chemotherapy, Ehrlich believed that he could manipulate atoxil in order to find, through controlled chemical reactions, new, more efficient side chains.

In 1909, together with one of his most brilliant assistants, the physician Sahachiro Hata, found one of the derivatives of atoxil, number 606, which proved to be able to cure syphilis in laboratory animals.

This product, which was given the trade name of Salvarsan, was announced as the first drug capable of treating the disease in 1910.

In 1908 he received the Nobel Prize for medicine, for

his theory of immunity. The prize was shared with the Russian Elie Metchnikoff, who developed studies on phagocytosis, the organism's basic defense mechanism.

Ehrlich was also the founder of hematology. He classified the leukocytes according to the presence or not of granules; differentiated leukemias; has shown that leukocytosis is a bone marrow response to infections and other stimuli; studied aplastic anemia and provided the basis for the cytochemical differentiation of the various cells involved with blood.

His work with antimicrobial dyes was a precursor to the discovery of sulfas, three decades later, by Gerhard Domagk.

He died in 1915, and few did as much for the development of medicine. Paul Ehrlich was, without a doubt, one of the greatest geniuses of humanity.

Marie Curie (A great scientist)

"Humanity needs dreamers, for whom the disinterested development of their work is so captivating that it is impossible for them to devote any attention to their personal benefit", said Marie Curie, who together with her husband, Pierre, isolated the radio , chemical element extracted from uraninite, with powerful radioactive capacity.

For their discovery, Pierre and Marie Curie received the 1903 Nobel Prize in physics. In 1906 Pierre died run over by a carriage. Marie continued to work on her research, and later came to receive the Nobel Prize in chemistry.

Despite all her ability, and despite having received so many awards, the French Academy of Sciences vetoed her as a partner, due to her female condition.

Her investigations were continued by one of her daughters, Irène Curie Joliot, who along with her husband, Frédéric Joliot, discovered that radioactivity could be induced in some normal atoms through the formation of isotopes.

In 1935, the Joliot couple also received the Nobel Prize in chemistry.

Among the developments of the discoveries of this brilliant family, we can mention the radiotherapy of tumors and the development of marked or radioactive substances, used for the diagnosis of diseases (such as radioimmunoassay).

Oswaldo Cruz (Our greatest sanitarian)

"From the first day we were able to admire the enchanting panorama that we see when we look into the eyepiece of a microscope, on whose platinum is a preparation; since we saw, with the help of this wonderful instrument, the numerous living beings that populate a drop of water; since we learned to cope, to handle with the microscope, the idea that our intellectual efforts from now on would converge so that we educate ourselves, specialize in a science that relies on microscopy, has taken root in our spirit". This is how Oswaldo

Gonçalves Cruz expressed himself, in the first paragraph of his thesis for the conclusion of the medical course, *The microbial transmission by waters,* in 1893.

Son of a doctor, Dr. Bento Gonçalves Cruz, for whom he had great admiration, Oswaldo Cruz lost his father the day he presented his thesis to the faculty.

He stayed in Rio de Janeiro for three years, working in a laboratory received as a wedding gift from his father-in-law.

In 1896 he traveled to Paris, together with his family. He attends the Pasteur Institute, where he improves his knowledge of bacteriology. He also does an internship in the urology service of Prof. Félix Guyon. He remains in France for three years.

After returning to Brazil, in October 1899, he was invited by the Minister of Health to, together with Adolfo Lutz and Vital Brazil, investigate the origin of an epidemic that was occurring in Santos. There were suspicions that it could be bubonic plague.

His report, sent on November 12, concluded that it was indeed a plague. After Santos, the epidemic spread to S. Paulo, Rio de Janeiro, Niterói and other cities in the country.

In Rio, the first case was diagnosed on January 7, 1900. It became an endemic disease, and in December 1905, 2,401 people died of this disease in the country's capital.

The measures taken by Oswaldo Cruz to combat this and other Brazilian endemics were presented in a report made at the 3rd International Sanitary Convention, held in Mexico City, in 1907, as follows:

Yellow fever - campaign against the vector (Aedes aegypti), through a force made up of a medical inspector, ten auxiliary inspectors, seventy-five medical students and a thousand health guards.

The staff was divided into three groups in charge of:

    1.   Isolation of patients and fumigation of houses.
    2.   Systematic elimination of mosquitoes, drying out temporary water deposits or throwing oil mixed with creoline on the ponds, or by means of fish that ate the mosquito larvae.
    3.   Protection of cisterns and other water sources.
    4.   Inspection of medical prescriptions, death verification and medical surveillance of non-immune people residing in outbreaks.

Bubonic plague - bactericidal and parasiticidal disinfection by means of phenols and cresols, aiming at the destruction of the bacillus and the transmitting flea (Pulex cheops), by monitoring households or by communicating with those interested.

In this disinfection, the solutions were used at an elevated temperature, and the floors were raised for complete disinfection.

The war against the rat was another measure taken and made by waterproofing the soil of all the houses neighboring the outbreaks and by systematic hunting for rodents.

The preventive inoculation of the antipestous serum was done when allowed. The serum was produced by the Instituto Manguinhos.

The systematic and indistinct isolation of all patients in a hospital, and the disinfection of the objects they handled, completed the measures used.

Malaria - war on mosquitoes in cities and clinical prophylaxis with quinine for three days in places with the highest incidence of the disease.

Just to have an idea of the yellow fever epidemic in Rio de Janeiro at that time, suffice it to say that in the year 1892 there were 4,312 deaths from the disease and, in 1909, after the measures taken by Oswaldo Cruz, there were no more case.

As for smallpox, it tried to implant mandatory vaccination in our country, but failed due to the strong popular reaction and the way vaccination was regulated.

He directed the Instituto Manguinhos, which in 1908 was renamed Instituto Oswaldo Cruz.

In 1912 he was elected to the Brazilian Academy of Letters, taking the place of the poet Raimundo Correia.

Oswaldo Cruz died in 1917, but he left as his main legacy the largest research institute in the country, an international reference as an institution focused on research and development in the area of public health.

The vaccine revolt

In Rio de Janeiro, in June 1904 alone, at the Hospital de S. Sebastião alone, over 1800 cases of hospitalization for smallpox had been reported.

In Brazil there were several endemic outbreaks of the disease and this caused great concern for the authorities, in addition to considerable losses for the country's economy.

A bill that mandated smallpox vaccination was then presented to Congress by Alagoas senator Manuel José Duarte.

Approved four months later, the regulation of mandatory vaccination, developed by Osvaldo Cruz and published on November 9, 1904, was what triggered the popular revolt.

As it is a considerably modest moral society, exposure by strangers to the intimate parts of the body of their women, mothers and daughters caused, in many people, great revolt and indignation.

Since there was no concern to raise awareness and prepare the population psychologically, from whom only total submission was expected, the revolt is a beautiful example of how a vaccination campaign should not be carried out.

The revolt began the day after the publication of the rules for the application of the vaccine and ended only on November 16, with the government revoking its mandatory nature.

In the period of the revolt, there were numerous conflicts between the popular - especially those from the poorest strata - and the police force. Even the Army and Navy participated in the repression.

At the end of the conflict, 23 people were killed, as well as 90 wounded and several people were arrested and banned to Acre.

Carlos Chagas (American trypanosomiasis)

Carlos Ribeiro Justiniano Chagas, first of the four children of José Justinano Chagas and Mariana Cândida Ribeiro Chagas, was born on July 9, 1878, at Fazenda Bom Retiro, near Oliveira, Minas Gerais.

Orphaned by a father at the age of four, Chagas spent his childhood on another family farm in Juiz de Fora, where his mother managed the cultivation of coffee.

Living with her maternal uncles - two lawyers and a doctor - made her, from an early age, express a desire to advance in her studies, with a special interest in medicine.

In 1897, he enrolled at the Faculty of Medicine, in Rio de Janeiro.

In 1902, he sought the then director of the Manguinhos Institute, Dr. Oswaldo Cruz, so that he could develop his doctoral thesis in medicine there, on hematological studies of malaria.

With the endorsement of the director, in two years he concluded his thesis.

Impressed with the work capacity and scientific knowledge shown by the young doctor, Oswaldo Cruz invited him, in 1903, to work in Manguinhos.

In July 1904, he married Íris Lobo, daughter of the Minas Gerais senator, Fernando Lobo, and from this union Evandro Chagas (1905) and Carlos Chagas Filho (1910) were born, both of whom became important scientists.

From 1907, Carlos Chagas started to develop research together with Cruz, in addition to other great national and foreign scientists, such as Arthur Neiva, Rocha Lima, Gustav Giemsa, von Prowazeck and Max Hartmann, this a great specialist in protozoa, who had a lot of importance in the scientific development of the young doctor.

In 1909, at the request of Oswaldo Cruz, he left for the interior to investigate an outbreak of malaria that was hampering the construction works of the Central Railway of Brazil, in a section near Pirapora, Minas Gerais, in a village called Lassance.

In this place, in addition to malaria, Chagas encounters a new, very frequent disease, where the affected people complained of a discomfort in the chest, and had arrhythmias, signs of heart failure, in addition to sudden death.

In addition to fighting the malaria outbreak, Chagas looked into the investigation of this new disease, when he learned from one of the railroad engineers that in the simple houses of the region's inhabitants (mud houses with many cracks, where insects hid), there were a lot of blood-sucking insects.

At night, these insects stung the open area of people's bodies, usually the face, which is why they were known as "barbers".

Examining the digestive tract of these insects, Chagas found a new type of protozoan, which had characteristics different from all the others he knew.

He then began to research the possible relationship between this microorganism and the disease he had just met.

On October 26, 1910, the National Academy of Medicine heard Carlos Chagas talk about American trypanosomiasis. From this disease, he was the discoverer of the etiologic agent, Trypanosoma cruzi; of the vector, Triatoma infestans; and the characteristics of the disease, both in its acute and chronic form. This is, to this day, an exceptional case in the history of medicine.

In 1917, with the death of Oswaldo Cruz, Chagas assumed the direction of the Instituto de Manguinhos, a position in which he would remain for the rest of his life.

In 1919, he was appointed to the General Directorate of Public Health, which, months later, would become the National Department of Public Health, with Chagas being its director from 1920 to 1926.

In 1923, he founded, in Rio de Janeiro, the Anna Nery School of Nursing and in 1926, he organized the Special Course in Public Health as a specialization at the Faculty of Medicine of Rio de Janeiro, which represented a milestone in the creation of the sanitary career in our parents.

It is estimated that there are currently, in Brazil, around 3.5 million people infected by the agent of the disease discovered by Carlos Chagas.

Because it is a disease with strong economic and social involvement, its control will only be effectively achieved when the rural population of our country comes to have better living conditions. Good quality houses and greater control of the transmitting agents (barbers) through the use of insecticides more efficient than DDT, for which there is already a lot of resistance, is essential. In addition, control of blood quality is critical to avoid transmission through transfusion, as may occur if the donor has the disease.

Recently, cases of transmission of the disease through the ingestion of contaminated food (sugarcane juice, açaí, etc.) have also been described, which can be explained by the fact that when the contaminated insect is crushed during milling, it releases thousands of protozoa from its intestine and that remain viable for several hours, thus being able to penetrate the human organism through the intestinal tract when ingested with some product.

Juliano Moreira (The new Brazilian psychiatric model)

Juliano Moreira was born in Salvador, in 1873, and died in Rio de Janeiro, in 1933. The contribution of this Afro-descendant doctor to the development of Brazilian psychiatry was significant, according to several studies published in the country and abroad[84].

Before him, mental illness is viewed in a prejudiced manner, where the moral criterion is emphasized over the illness itself, that is, the notion of behavior disorder prevails over the importance of intellectual disorder as an element that formulates psychopathology.

The mental disease in Brazil was described from symptoms, showing still the focus of Pinel and Esquirol and considering the existence of different forms of madness: dementia and idiocy would be characterized by unreason; while the delusions and disorders of intelligence due to the predominance of passions and which would represent monomanias. These would be determined by a partial injury of intelligence, by affectivity, thus constituting a behavior disorder.

Alienation being considered as a behavior disorder

would imply aiming at re-educating the alienated, that is, the orientation of a treatment should be eminently moral.

This idea prevails over the construction of asylums of the nineteenth century and were spaces designed to isolate the alienated environmental contributor to the development of their vices, besides allowing the presence of the doctor, it would be important patient recovery factor for its ability to impose a reorganization of your way of thinking and behaving.

The concept of degeneration acting on the psychological was a consequence mainly of the knowledge that certain pathologies - epilepsy, syphilis, chemical dependence - could trigger a psychopathology.

In addition to this, the issue of heredity can be added, which was seen as an important contributing factor for degeneration, in addition to the racial issue, due to the fact that at the time it was common to confuse race with social class, without taking into account differentiated access to education and, consequently, to a better quality of life of those who had greater purchasing power and came from a higher social level.

In 1903 Juliano Moreira began a new administration at the National Hospital for Alienated Persons, in Rio de Janeiro, treated until then as a detention facility for the insane, with no adequate treatment, discipline or even inspection.

Thereafter, conducted a comprehensive reform in the hospital and that only was concluded the following year.

Among the various modifications made, may cite new amenities include kitchen, laundry and the morgue; an electricity generator designed to supply constant energy to the hospice; one the medical library and one the sick ; and new pavilions were also built (one for children, another for epileptics and sex-separated wards for patients with intercurrent infectious diseases).

The school pavilion, dedicated exclusively to children, offered specialized treatment different from that given to adults . It had a room with gym equipment, a course for school education, appropriate beds and a geometric garden, for better knowledge of shapes and relief.

A pathological anatomy laboratory, an experimental psychology office and a permanent surgical service were also created.

There was yet another pavilion built to carry out trades, understood as tools for disciplining and treating. The space housed blacksmithing and firefighter workshops; electrical mechanics; carpentry and joinery; typography and binding; shoe store; bedding; broom and painting ; tapestry; flower making and sewing. All of this contributed to giving the mentally ill a more dignified and efficient treatment, which was not the norm until then.

Juliano Moreira was also responsible for initiating studies in Brazil on epilepsy, alcoholism and syphilis as possible causes of delusions that could lead to madness and, as a result, as relevant causes of delinquency and crime. With his work, he also contributed to the fight against racism, at the time very common in our country.

Based on Kraepelin's theory - a German psychiatry that was important for the development of modern psychiatry - , Juliano Moreira considers the difference between dementia and paranoia, seen as a result of the individual's inability to adapt to the social, maintaining a primitive egocentrism. Mental health goes then to be defined by the man's behavior notion of balance with the social environment, in frank opposition to previous view that was eminently moral.

The discovery of insulin

In 1869, a German medical student, named Paul Langerhans, observed that in the pancreas there were two types of cells, acinar cells, which secrete digestive enzymes, and cells clustered on islands or islets, which suggested a possible new function for them.

The first reports of pancreas removal and the development of diabetes mellitus were recorded by von Mering and Minkowski, in an article published in 1889. However, it was only in 1922 that a work published by Frederick G. Banting reported the satisfactory result obtained with the treatment of seven diabetic patients by the use of pancreatic extract, containing a substance called - by Banting - insulin, due to the location of the hormone-producing cells. To help him discover insulin, Banting was supported by a 4th year medical student from Toronto, named Charles Best.

Banting believed that he could only extract the hormone involved in diabetes if it prevented its degradation by the proteolytic action of pancreatic juice, which was released through the organ's ducts. He then ligated the ducts, which led to the subsequent degeneration of the acinar tissues, leaving the islet cells intact. He subsequently extracted the pancreatic extract with alcohol and acid, which has been shown to be effective in reducing blood glucose levels.

The first patient treated by them was Leonard Thompson, a 14-year-old boy, who arrived at Toronto General Hospital with a blood glucose of 500 mg% (the normal rate ranges from 70 to 99 mg%) and with a daily diuresis of 3 to 5 liters. Despite undergoing a strict diet (450 kcal per day), his diabetes was totally out of control and his death was imminent. After the administration of Banting and Best extracts, there was a considerable clinical and laboratory change. His blood glucose rose to levels close to 100 mg% and the boy had a significant improvement in health. The suspension of treatment, on the other hand, reversed the entire process, which demonstrated the importance of administering the new type of treatment.

Subsequently, Banting obtained the adhesion of the professor of physiology, Macleod, which led to the purification and greater production of the hormone. In 1923, Banting and Macleod shared the Nobel Prize in Medicine and Physiology. Banting announced that he would share his share with Best, out of his contribution to the initial research on the discovery of insulin.

In 1953, Frederick Sanger was able to determine the complete sequence of the insulin molecule, having received the Nobel Prize for chemistry in 1958.

Fleming (The discovery of penicillin)

Alexander Fleming was born in Scotland in 1881. He

graduated in medicine and in 1922 he discovered that in secretions, such as nasal mucus, saliva and tears, there was an enzyme that destroyed bacteria, which he called lysozyme.

In 1928, while studying variants of a bacterium called staphylococcus, after leaving a plaque several days on the bench in his laboratory at St. Mary's Hospital in London, he observed the presence of a contaminating fungus, the species Penicillium notatum.

The interesting fact, which caught his attention, was a halo of inhibition of bacterial growth around the colony of the fungus.

From the knowledge he had acquired while studying lysozyme, Fleming believed that this inhibition would be a consequence of some type of similar substance, produced by Penicillium.

He then started to work with the fungus in culture broth, and was able to verify that it produced a substance that caused a strong inhibition in the growth of several microbes. As the fungus belonged to the genus Penicillium, it gave this substance the name of penicillin.

In 1929, Fleming published the first scientific paper on penicillin, but only in 1940 - with the support of researchers Howard Florey and Ernst Chain - was it possible to produce penicillin in its most purified form.

In one test, Florey and Chain injected fifty mice with a lethal dose of a bacterium, streptococcus. Twenty-five animals were injected with penicillin every three hours, for a period of 45 hours. At the end of ten days, 24 of the 25 treated mice had survived. On the other hand, all 25 control mice, who did not receive the antibiotic, died.

These results were published in August 1940 in the Lancet magazine and were received with great enthusiasm by everyone.

A new stage in the health sciences was inaugurated. For their work on the development of penicillin, Fleming, Florey and Chain received the Nobel Prize in medicine in 1945.

Freud and the creation of psychoanalysis

Psychoanalysis came to fill a space that emerged after the great development obtained by neurology and psychiatry during the 19th century.

The term psychoanalysis is related to an investigation method for studying the most intimate and hidden regions of the spirit; to a theory that is elaborated with the results of this analysis and to a technique that aims to adopt the analytical method in the treatment of imbalances of the mind.

Psychoanalysis is the only science that deeply exercises self-reflection, or reflection on the motivations of a subconscious, personal and emotional order that go, insensibly, conditioning knowledge and forming the personality of each one.

Pinel, at the end of the 18th century, had implemented major changes in the treatment of mental illnesses with his hospital reform. The set of non-physical measures that preserved and morally improved the mentally ill, in addition to avoiding frequent iatrogenies, constituted the core of these reforms.

Psychotherapy has a more scientific character from the schools of Nancy, under the command of Hippolyte Bernheim (1840-1919) and Paris, with Jean Martin Charcot (1825-1893). French psychiatry was divided between these two schools, which differed on some issues, such as those concerning hysteria and the use of hypnosis as a semiotic medium.

Charcot believed that the state of hypnosis was essentially the same as that of hysteria, deducing that a person's ease in allowing himself to be suggested by hypnosis meant latent hysteria. Consequently, he doubted to attach any value to hypnotism for the treatment of mental disorders.

Bernheim, for his part, disagreed with Charcot's theories about hysteria and the correspondence between hypnosis and neurotic behavior.

Meanwhile, through the studies of Charles Bell, François Magendie, Brown-Séquard, Paul Broca and Claude Bernard, neurology and neurophysiology provided considerable support for the diagnosis and understanding of a series of diseases, previously little known and of pathophysiological basis foggy.

Sigmund Freud (1856-1939), born in Freiberg, a small town in Moravia, graduated in medicine in 1881 in Vienna. Then he studied in Paris, from 1885 to 1886, with Charcot from whom he learned the relationships between hysteria and sexuality. Charcot's thesis was that at the base of these cases there was always sexual trauma, that his memory was hidden by the minds of hysterics.

He later developed a technique with Austrian doctor Josef Breuer in which patients could discuss their emotional problems by free association. The procedure unleashed powerful forces, which dragged uncontrolled thoughts in the direction of the psychic conflict, eventually resolving the neurotic condition then existing. Breuer had thus created the cathartic method and discovered the intimate relationship between hysterical symptoms and certain childhood traumas. In the book they both published on hysteria in 1895, they highlighted the etiological significance of sexual life in neuroses.

According to his doctrine, the memory of past events plays an important role in people's lives and the mental conflicts often produced by such memories can be removed when brought to the surface (to the conscious). This if the conflict is properly understood through a long process of research from the unconscious, which has as one of its characteristics never to forget what happens to us.

Later, Freud broke with Breuer and began to further develop the method of free association of ideas. This leads him to the two foundations that form the basis of psychoanalysis, resistance (the defense mechanism that the patient presents when he feels that his repressed experiences are revealed) and transference (the emotional bond between the patient and the analyst).

In summary, it can also be said that psychoanalysis tries to understand the basis of human behavior based on three fundamental concepts:

> a) The existence of an unconscious mind, demonstrated through examples such as those provided by dreams, selective forgetfulness and post-hypnotic events.

b) Psychic determinism, which says that nothing happens by chance, or that all psychic events are determined by other facts or events.

c) The mechanism of repression, which prevents events that are too painful to arise from consciousness.

The Interpretation of Dreams is considered the foundation of psychoanalysis. Freud was the first researcher to transform the dream into an object of science. According to him, dreams are not products of chance, but contents of our unconscious trying to reach consciousness. Published in 1900, with a circulation of 600 copies, the book had only 351 units sold after two years of being published. Freud himself complained, in *History of the Psychoanalytic Movement*, that his book "was not even commented on in the specialized literature and, in the few cases in which this occurred, was criticized with compassionate superiority or with sarcasm".

While traditional psychotherapy seeks - through suggestion, persuasion or other repressive methods - to add something to modify the image of the personality, psychoanalysis tries to free the personality from what is preventing it from taking on its authentic form.

Following a model cited by Freud, traditional psychotherapy would correspond to painting an empty canvas in color, while psychoanalysis would act as the sculptor who worked the marble until the image hidden in it appeared.

The method that psychoanalysis uses is a form of communication, verbal and non-verbal, which allows the patient to rescue the psychological trauma that generated the neurotic process from his unconscious.

The analyst acts as a mirror, which only reflects what is shown to him. By discovering the unconscious and its laws, the analyzed person will be able to rescue elements of his personality that were asleep.

For Freud, human nature is not generous. The coexistence between men would depend on the internalization of the natural aggressiveness of the human being, with a deviation from the direction of the external object and its return to the individual.

According to Mac Lean[85], the human brain contains a more primitive part, the paleocephalus; an intermediate, the mesocephalus; and a more recently developed one, the cortex, which in humans is more developed than in other animals, being called the neocortex. The paleocephalus, heir to the reptilian brain, would be the source of aggression and drives. The mesocephalus, from the ancient mammals, would be linked to affectivity and long-term memory. The neocortex, on the other hand, would be the seat of the most elaborate thoughts and reasoning, characteristic of the human species. There is not always harmony between these three levels of mental complexity. Now one predominates, now another. The result of this eternal conflict is the average action of each person, throughout his existence.

We live under the influence of two basic drives, either tanatic and erotic, and renouncing them would develop our superego, or the basis of the moral instance that limits us. The human being must then accept the partial renunciation of the omnipotence of the drive in order to live socially. Psychic maturity would be the result of the gradual transition from mental functioning marked by pleasure (as in childhood narcissism) to another influenced by the reality principle, or the gradual transition to psychic maturity, where there is a maturation of the mind, with a larger space for altruism and gratitude.

Jonathan Lear, professor of Philosophy at the University of Chicago, maintains that psychoanalysis is essential to living in a democratic society, as it is a technique that allows obscure meanings and irrational motivations to reach the surface of consciousness and can be properly worked on. As a result, they may become less able to emerge in violent and incomprehensible forms, as they have happened countless times, when, for example, apparently normal individuals murder innocent people, who had nothing to do with their anxieties or frustrations. Or even when fanaticism serves as a justification for violent actions against others.

According to Freud, psychoanalysis lends itself only to the treatment of neuroses. Both emergency cases, suicidal tendencies in melancholy patients and psychoses are diseases that orbit the space of psychiatry.

Since its emergence, psychoanalysis has met with resistance in various sectors of society, receiving criticism caused by being a new science and also due to the very object of that science.

According to Freud, "psychoanalysis wants to raise the repressed psychic materials to the level of conscious recognition, and each man who judges him is himself someone who has such repressions and who may only keep them with great effort. Psychoanalysis arouses in these people the same resistance as in patients, and this resistance easily manages to put on an intellectual disguise and mobilize arguments, just as those brandished by our patients, when they revolt against the fundamental rule of analysis. Like the sick, our adversaries are also often characterized by a significant deterioration in their judgment, due to affective factors. There is the same resistance in these people as in the sick, the same arguments, affections disguised as reasons ".

Psychoanalysis is also combated for being a source of humiliation for human narcissism, for having demonstrated that we are influenced by uncontrollable aspects of our unconscious[86] , having repercussions similar to that which occurred after Copernicus showed that the Earth is not the center of the universe, and that Darwin restored man to the animal king[87].

The natural history of diseases

Soon after the start of bacteriology, there was a great expectation that diseases would be easily eliminated from the knowledge of their respective causes.

Over time, it was found that, in addition to the causative agent of each infection, there were several other factors that interacted for a given disease to develop.

Thus, the fact that a person, for example, comes into contact with the tuberculosis bacillus does not necessarily make him or her tuberculous.

Factors such as the presence or absence of malnutrition, housing conditions, frequent contact with patients with the disease, exposure to cold, or conditions related to the environment, also contribute significantly to whether or not tuberculosis, in the form of the disease.

This interaction - host / agent / environment - is valid for both infectious and parasitic diseases, as well as for other types of diseases.

Before a disease is detected clinically, it has to develop preliminary organic changes, only detectable through complementary exams. There is, therefore, a pre-clinical phase that precedes the clinical phase of the diseases.

The major consequence of knowing the natural history of diseases is the fact that, when trying to control or prevent a type of disease, one has to adopt a multifactorial approach and not aim only at controlling one of its causes, as is usually the case. think.

Medical education in the USA

The lack of legal regulations led the United States of America (USA) to have hundreds of medical schools during the 19th century. Several of them were veritable "diploma factories", graduating professionals with no qualifications.

With the creation of the American Medical Association (AMA), in 1847, an attempt was made to change this situation by trying to raise the level of the profession and preventing bad professionals and charlatans from continuing to act.

Abraham Flexner was born in Lousville, Kentucky, on November 13, 1866, the sixth child of European immigrants, and graduated in education in 1886 at John Hopkins University.

At the beginning of the 20th century, he completed his master's degree in education at Harvard.

In 1908 he published the book *The American College: A Criticism*, which earned him an invitation to work for the Carnegie Foundation, in a survey that examined the teaching conditions of medicine in the USA.

After two years of inspection visits, Flexner produced a report that marked the beginning of a radical reform movement in medical education in North America.

The report, *Medical Education in the United States and Canada*, was published in 1910, and recommended the reduction of the number of medical schools and the number of students, as there was a production of doctors that considerably exceeded the needs of the market.

According to him, 31 good medical schools could do a better job than the 155 schools of varying quality that he had visited during his research.

It was suggested that the transfer of the Carnegie Foundation's money should be made only to the best medical schools, according to the report. Proposals were also made to reform the curriculum of the colleges.

The main recommendations of the report consisted of the creation of departments, the creation of the basic cycle in science, the development of research within the scope of basic areas and the creation of teaching hospitals to be used as the main clinical training scenarios.

From 1913, when he started to act as secretary of the General Council of Education of the Rockefeller Foundation, Flexner obtained large philanthropic donations for the development of medical schools in the USA, which generated a contribution of resources in the order of 600 million dollars.

In 1930, schools were reduced to 76 institutions of high educational standards, which contributed to making medicine developed in the USA one of the best in the world.

The Rockefeller Foundation was instrumental in making university activities more professional. His performance was characterized by an emphasis on basic sciences, which occupied the center of research in the 1930s and 1940s.

In Brazil, its influence occurred mainly through financing, having been especially relevant at the Federal University of S. Paulo and Minas Gerais.

In 1964 alone, the Escola Paulista de Medicina (EPM) received US $ 716,000 from the Rockfeller Foundation, which contributed, three years later, to become the headquarters of the Regional Library of Medicine, better known as BIREME, through an agreement signed between the Pan American Health Organization, Ministry of Education, Ministry of Health and EPM.

BIREME was inspired by the American model institution, the National Library of Medicine (NLM), with access to the MEDLARS database, created and headquartered at NLM, access to the collection of journals from the same library and with the mission of developing integration between associated libraries in Latin America.

The first university in Brazil emerged during the government of Epitácio Pessoa, in the 1920s, when it brought together the Polytechnic School, the Faculty of Law and the School of Medicine of Rio de Janeiro. Then, the Federal University of Minas Gerais was created in 1927 and that of S. Paulo in 1934, which resulted from the incorporation of several faculties such as Law, Polytechnic, Medicine, Pharmacy and Dentistry, the Instituto de Education, Agriculture and Philosophy, Science and Letters.

The creation of universities was in line with the thinking of our intellectual elite who claimed their emergence in the country, aiming at higher education in an integrated way with society.

Most important diseases in the early 20th century

Yellow fever

It was first described in 1684 and, for more than two centuries, it caused a considerable loss of human life in much of the world.

For a long time it was believed to be the disease resulting from contaminated air, or *miasma*, which made it difficult to control the various epidemics that plagued countries in tropical regions.

Elucidation of transmission of yellow fever was made by Reed Mission, organized by the US Army Health Service, sent to Cuba on June 25, 1900 to investigate the etiology and the prevention of the disease. The group consisted of medical major Walter Reed, James Carrol, Jesse Lazear and Aristides Agramonte.

Reed, influenced by Cuban doctor Carlos Finlay, came to support the transmission will the virus pel the *Aedes aegypti*, ie the need for an intermediate host for the disease to establish itself.

On January 14, 1901 he published the work "The mosquito as an agent of the spread of yellow fever", in which he clearly defended the theory of arthropods in the transmission of yellow fever.

In Brazil, at the beginning of the 20th century, the disease also caused several epidemics in Santos and in the interior of the State of S. Paulo. After the dissemination of Reed's work, Emílio Ribas, director of the São Paulo Health Service since 1898, also started to support the theory of the transmission of the disease by the mosquito.

Due to the rejection of this theory by a still considerable number of Brazilian doctors, Emílio Ribas decided to repeat some of the experiments that had been carried out in Cuba by the Reed Mission.

Together, among others with Adolfo Lutz, he underwent experimental inoculation by infected mosquitoes. Of the six people bitten, three acquired the disease, one with a severe form.

He also had another experiment that consisted of exposing some volunteers to contact with clothes infected by patients, in an indoor environment and without mosquitoes. In this case, no volunteers were infected.

It proved in this way that the transmission of the virus was due to the mosquito and not to contact with patients or materials contaminated by them.

His experiences were presented at the 5th Brazilian Congress of Medicine and Surgery, held in Rio de Janeiro in 1903 and chaired by Oswaldo Cruz.

The virus was isolated in 1927, and the yellow fever vaccine began to be used in 1934.

Because it has wild reservoirs, such as some species of monkeys, in addition to transmitting mosquitoes, the disease cannot be extinguished in forests, as in the Amazon and in parts of Africa and tropical Asia.

Unimmunized people who enter areas of reservoirs of the disease may acquire the disease, which leads to severe hepatitis and kidney failure, with a high mortality rate.

The flu

Since the 16th century, epidemics of febrile respiratory diseases have been described every three years. The high rate of attack, the explosive nature of the epidemics and the frequency of coughs, chills, generalized pain and runny nose accompanying the symptoms, suggest that it was influenza outbreaks, a disease caused mainly by influenza A and B viruses.

The origin of the name influenza is attributed to Italian doctors and would be a consequence of the doctrines prevalent in the beginning of the modern era, which linked physical disorders to astrological phenomena, such as the relationship that was made between the appearance of epidemics and the appearance of comets and meteors, or even to volcanic eruptions or even sudden weather changes. Thus, everything that happened on our planet would be due to the influence of the stars, which motivated the name given to the disease.

The last influenza pandemic of the 19th century, in 1889 and 1890, was the first during the bacteriological era. Soon after, in 1892, the German bacteriologist Richard Pfeiffer claimed to have found, in samples taken from the respiratory tract of patients, a bacterium he had named as *Haemophilus influenzae*. Wrongly, Pfeiffer considered the microbe as the cause of the flu. However, the influenza virus was not discovered until 1933. It is now known that the bacillus discovered by Pfeiffer causes only one of several types of acute bacterial pneumonias.

Influenza is a viral disease that was possibly acquired through human contact with domesticated animals, such as birds and pigs.

In terms of morbidity and mortality, none of the pandemics came close to what occurred in 1918 and 1919, known as the Spanish flu, when about 40 to 100 million people died worldwide.

As the therapeutic and preventive resources at that time were restricted to quarantine and isolation, little can be done to prevent the spread of the disease, as well as its high lethality rates.

Subsequent serological studies, carried out in the USA, showed that the population most affected in this pandemic was 5 to 15 years old.

The same age group was also the most affected in the 1957 pandemic, originating in China, which was caused by the influenza virus type A, serotype H2 N2 (subtypes of the hemagglutinin and neuraminidase antigens that serve to typify influenza viruses).

The virus was further isolated from pigs in China, suggesting that the transmission to humans was from domestic animal breeding in Asia.

Because the flu virus to be in always changing through frequent mutations, several virology laboratories in different countries exert constant vigilance in order to detect any appearance of a new type of these microbes. If this occurs, health authorities should be notified immediately, so that prophylactic measures can be implemented in a short period of time in order to prevent a rapid spread of the disease.

In 2003 a new type of virus scared the world. Coronaviruses were responsible for Severe Acute Respiratory Syndrome (SARS), which had a mortality rate of up to 50% in some older age groups. It was considered the first pandemic of the 21st century, demonstrating once again the need for constant control of viruses that cause respiratory diseases, similar to what is already done with influenza viruses.

In 2009, a new pandemic arose due to the same A / H1N1 virus, a descendant of the person responsible for the pandemic of the early 20th century, and which has worried health authorities around the world.

According to data from the World Health Organization, until the beginning of November 2009, there were 503 thousand cases of pandemic influenza in the different continents, with just over six thousand deaths and a lethality of 1.2%.

In Brazil, in the same period, there were 22,500 cases with 1,500 deaths, that is, a lethality close to 7%.

The main risk groups - and the ones most subject to complications due to this new pandemic - were the extremes of age (less than two years and over sixty), pregnant women, smokers and people with chronic diseases, especially those of origin pulmonary, cardiovascular and immunosuppressive.

Between the 1st A / H1N1 virus pandemic and the current one there are some differences that could explain the lower lethality in the current one:

- When the first pandemic occurred, there was no awareness in the international community that the threat could be so significant. In this case, the 1st epidemic due to its impact on morbidity and mortality was unprecedented in human history.

- There was also no global epidemiological surveillance system for influenza viruses at the time of the 1st pandemic. WHO was not created until 1948.

- Today, vaccines, antivirals and antibiotics are available, which significantly contributes to reducing morbidity and mortality from influenza viruses. In addition, there are currently laboratory tests for a quick and accurate diagnosis, providing faster and more efficient treatment and isolation measures, also contributing to limit the spread of the disease.

- There is no conflict like World War I, which contributed significantly to a greater and faster spread of the virus. Studies suggest that the pandemic strain originated from a rural area of the state of Kansas, then spread to the USA with the mobilization by World War I and then spread to Europe together with the American Expeditionary Force.

The contemporary art of cure

Philosophers cannot isolate themselves against science. It not only greatly expanded and transformed our view of life and the universe, but it also revolutionized the rules by which the intellect operates.

Claude Lévi-Strauss

The discovery of the genetic code

In 1868, the Swiss physician Miescher described the first report of nucleoproteins from cells obtained from surgical bandages discarded from a hospital. Later, he isolated a similar substance from salmon sperm, and showed that the nucleoprotein consisted of a basic protein (protamine) and a nucleic acid.

Later, Levene, a Russian chemist based in the USA,

discovered, in 1909, that there were two types of nucleic acid, DNA (deoxyribonucleic acid) and RNA (ribonucleic acid). He thought, however, that it was the protein molecules that stored genetic information in the chromosomes of cells.

It was the work of an English bacteriologist, Frederick Griffith, who in 1928, working with pneumococci, helped to elucidate the problem. He realized that an unknown substance, obtained from dead bacteria, was able to penetrate other living microbes and transfer characteristics of the dead variety to the living variety.

In 1944, another bacteriologist, Oswald Avery, demonstrated that it was DNA, not protein or RNA, that was responsible for the genetic transformation of bacteria. While DNA consists of the genetic material responsible for heredity, RNA makes our cells follow the orders contained in DNA perfectly.

Both DNA and RNA are made up of sugars (deoxyribose or ribose) and nitrogenous bases such as adenine, guanine, cytosine, thymine and uracil (this only exists in RNA). DNA has a double strand, while RNA has a single strand, like a strand.

The way in which these substances came together, forming the molecule of each nucleic acid, was discovered by Watson and Crick, in 1953, when they demonstrated that the DNA strands are arranged in an antiparallel way and the bases are paired along the entire length, forming a double helix. The two tapes are matched by means of nitrogenous bases. Adenine pairs with thymine and cytosine with guanine.

In addition to Watson and Crick, they also developed works in this area Maurice Wilkins (with whom they shared the Nobel Prize in 1962) and Rosalind Franklin. Because he died prematurely, at 37, Franklin did not come to be awarded the Nobel Prize along with the others. His studies of

X-ray diffraction allowed to elucidate the helical structure of DNA. His photograph of No. 51, of the hydrated form of the molecule, is what led Watson and Crick to correctly complete their construction of the DNA molecule.

In 1964, the genetic code was deciphered by three biochemists from the *National Institute of Health* , MW Nirenberg, JH Mathaei and P. Leder. They synthesized small molecules of RNA, of known composition, and observed which amino acids were incorporated in the formation of proteins. By testing the 64 possibilities of the four nitrogenous RNA bases, combined in groups of three, they were able to identify the exact code for each amino acid.

The importance of this knowledge in the replication of DNA, and in the synthesis of RNA of complementary sequences, was soon recognized.

The language in which the genetic information is read and executed was discovered.

In the near future, it is likely that the genome will become the main source of information for diagnoses and treatments to be determined, just as gene therapy can become a reality capable of eliminating a series of diseases that are still responsible for today. cause many deaths and suffering.

New technologies and the evolution of health sciences

From the second half of the twentieth century, a series of new technologies was added to the health sciences, causing a new world of possibilities for patient care to be introduced in clinical and surgical practice.

Laboratory medicine, which had its first book *Laboratory diagnosis for the practioner* published in 1906, by the American James C. Todd, has considerable development today. This can be seen through the inclusion of new methodologies, such as immunoenzymatic and immunochemical assays, polymerase chain reactions, blood cell subpopulation counts, in addition to hundreds of biochemical tests and screening for various types of diseases. Sensitivity tests to antimicrobials, previously restricted to bacteria, can now also be performed for other types of microorganisms, such as fungi and viruses.

In 1911, the Dutchman Willem Einthoven, developed the first device capable of recording the electrical activity of the heart, which allows the emergence of a new approach in the investigation of cardiovascular diseases.

Later, in 1924, the German Hans Berger, succeeded in registering, in a rudimentary way and for the first time, electrical waves emitted by a person's brain, starting from there the development of the electroencephalogram (EEG). However, he was unaware of the physical and technical bases of what he had found.

Only with the support of two British electrophysiologists, Edgar Adrian and BH Mathews, who, in 1934, confirmed Berger's findings, was it possible for international recognition of the findings of encephalography in a forum in 1937.

Then, new types of treatment are added to clinical and surgical practice, allowing more and more people to be cured of various types of illnesses considered serious, previously responsible for high levels of mortality rates.

When Dr. Christian Barnard, in 1967, at the Groote

Schuur Hospital in Cape Town, South Africa, performed the first heart transplant, there were still great difficulties in controlling the risk of rejection. With the evolution of pharmacology and the introduction of new drugs, such as cyclosporine, this risk has been controlled and today we are able to perform transplants of various types of organs, such as those of the heart, lung, kidney, bones, pancreas, liver and marrow bone.

With the introduction of stem cell research, organ rejection problems will soon disappear or become much less important than they are today.

In 1978, doctors Patrick Steptoe and Robert Edwards announced the birth of Louise Brown, the first baby conceived by the "in vitro" fertilization technique, outside the womb. From then on, humanity started to rely on new assisted reproduction techniques, which came to considerably improve the expectations of couples with infertility problems, which occurs around 15% of the world population.

Surgical specialties have been developing over the past 50 years. Today myocardial revascularization surgeries are performed in several hospitals around the world, using less and less invasive techniques. This has also occurred with other surgical specialties, which have increasingly used endoscopic surgeries, with less complications and less postoperative time.

Computer science and the evolution of diagnostic imaging have moved us from the era of X-rays to another where new equipment has emerged, much more advanced, such as those that allowed the development of much more sophisticated and sensitive exams. Ultrasound, scintigraphy, helical tomography and magnetic resonance imaging currently allow a level of diagnostic possibilities never before imagined by doctors in the past.

Ethics in scientific research

The Nazi theory - and that of other radical right-wing groups - of the supremacy of the "Aryan race", proved to be totally false with scientific evolution.

Recent genetic studies show that the physical characteristics responsible for the differences in skin color are expressed in less than ten genes, that is, an insignificant percentage in relation to about 25 thousand genes that make up the human genome.

Furthermore, according to paleoanthropology, all human beings are descended from the same African population, which, formed about 100 to 200 thousand years ago, emigrated to other continents[88].

As a result, skin color is a mere evolutionary adaptation to different levels of ultraviolet radiation, with no justification for speaking of race as something that can separate us.

In addition to Nazi experiments with prisoners of war, racial and political persecutions that horrified humanity so much, several researches have been carried out throughout history without great ethical concerns.

In 1947, an international court met in the city of Nuremberg, Germany, where Nazi doctors responsible for various crimes against humanity were tried.

In addition to the trial, a set of ethical guidelines for clinical research was developed, which became known as the Nuremberg Code. Despite being known to all, the ethical guidelines contained in the code were not always able to sensitize some researchers.

In the United States of America, for example, there was a famous research on the development of syphilis, which started in 1932 and ended in the 70s. It became known as "Tuskegee's research", because it is the name of the location in Alabama where lived the community object of the experience.

During the research period 408 patients, all black and poor, were kept untreated, and another 192 (non-syphilitic) were used as a control group. None were alerted that they were being tested. On the contrary, they informed them that they would receive "free special treatment".

The 41-year study led to the publication of 13 scientific papers. In one of these papers published in 1954, the authors demonstrated that mortality among untreated syphilitic patients was higher than among presumably non-syphilitic patients, in addition to having their disease worsened over the years.

The patients continued to receive no treatment, despite the fact that penicillin has been in use since the 1940s. The scientific community itself, inexplicably, was silent about the ethical issues surrounding this research.

The study was only interrupted in 1972, when it was denounced by a Washington Star journalist.

In June 1964, during the 18th General Assembly of the World Medical Association, held in Finland, the Declaration of Helsinki was released. Even today, it is considered the most important ethical reference for the regulation of medical research involving human beings, basically meaning the acceptance, by medical entities all over the world, of the precepts established by the Nuremberg Code.

In Brazil, the first standards for research on human beings were initially established by Resolution No. 1 of June 18, 1988, of the National Health Council, of the Ministry of Health. The national standards had the character of orientation and awareness of society about the importance of ethics in science. All research on human beings should be submitted, still in the design phase, to an ethics committee, recommended Resolution 1/88.

On October 10, 1996, other standards came into force, after their publication in the Federal Official Gazette, through Resolution No. 196 of the National Health Council.

It incorporates the four basic references of bioethics: autonomy or freedom (the subjects of the experiments must give their free and fully informed consent), non-maleficence, beneficence and justice. Similar to Resolution No. 1, all research involving human subjects must be submitted to the appreciation of a research ethics committee.

If it is not possible to set up a committee of its own, the institution where the research is to be carried out (or the main researcher) must submit the project to the committee of another institution. The project must contain an adhesion term in which each person freely and consciously consents to participate in the research. Such requirements apply to any type of study, regardless of the method used.

However, despite all these recommendations, there are still ethical deviations in scientific research carried out in several countries, including Brazil. One of the main problems lies in the use of a placebo, or in the use of a false medication, without the presence of an active ingredient, which is used to neutralize a possible improvement of a certain disease just for psychological reasons or suggestion.

According to the Declaration of Helsinki, placebo could only be used when there was no effective treatment for the disease. This does not always happen, as when several studies are presented in which the placebo is used in diseases such as hypertension, migraine and depression, among others. In these cases, the use of placebo is totally unjustified, since there are several drugs of recognized efficacy for the treatment of these diseases.

Recent data show that our country is one of the countries that most use human volunteers in clinical research. According to the National Research Ethics Commission (CONEP), in 2001 alone, 645 thousand Brazilians participated in research, most of them using drugs from foreign laboratories. Almost all of these people were poor patients, served by the public health system.

A glance at history

According to Hobsbawn (*On History,* 1997), modern science systematically and deliberately neglects historical experience. The current model is to expect a definitive answer, on any subject, from computers increasingly resembling an ethereal being, from whom nothing is expected but infallibility.

Furthermore, scientific evolution has led the current civilization to increasingly believe in scientific knowledge and technology, considering it even capable of replacing or even surpassing God.[89].

One of the aims of historical materialism was to bring history closer to the social sciences, avoiding the exaggerated simplifications of positivism. According to the founder of historical materialism, societies are systems of relationships between human beings, with a fundamental relationship between the social being and consciousness.

Thus, we cannot develop a health professional without providing training supported by the social sciences. The importance of the lack of this view can be exemplified by the neglect with which public health is still treated in Brazil. This can be proven by observing diseases that were previously apparently controlled, such as yellow fever, cholera, leprosy and tuberculosis, returning to the headlines again, in addition to the emergence of new endemic diseases, such as dengue and AIDS.

This situation can be attributed to several factors, but also to the forgetfulness of the sanitary history of civilization. What was a priority in the past, has become no longer in the present, such as the campaigns developed by Oswaldo Cruz to combat the yellow fever vector, at the beginning of the 20th century. The consequences have a high economic and social cost.

Regarding the potential of nations, today mineral resources are not valued as much as they were in the past, but human capital, which is the major driver of the development of a state. How can we think about great transformations, if our people continue to be at the mercy of the same diseases and limitations, long abolished in developed countries?

On the other hand, the 20th century produced major changes and technological innovations. We started to live with a degree of comfort, technology and facilities that our ancestors never imagined.

But have we really changed so much?

Hobsbawn teaches us that, despite being taller and heavier than our ancestors, who lived in the caves, biologically and emotionally the man is almost the same.

We are still selfish, envious and unlikely to think of humanity as one big family.

Perhaps we can dream, in the future, of a world without borders, and with greater solidarity, in which there is no hunger, misery, war, disease or any other type of suffering for all the inhabitants of this blue planet, the first home of the human being in the universe. infinite.

The chronic diseases

With regard to chronic non-communicable diseases, Robert Koch's postulates are no longer adequate.

For this group of diseases, where the causes are multiple, differently from infectious diseases, the support of modern epidemiology and statistics has become essential.

After the introduction of antimicrobials, that is, from the 1940s, the scourge of infectious diseases was replaced by an increasing number of deaths due to cardiovascular diseases, such as arterial hypertension, coronary atherosclerotic disease and stroke.

These diseases were the main cause of mortality in developed countries like the USA, making the average life expectancy not to exceed 45 years.

In addition, there were no adequate treatments for these diseases, both for chronic and acute events, and little is known about the determining factors for the evolution of these diseases.

One fact that also contributed to a greater interest in the study of this group of diseases was the premature death of President Franklin D. Roosevelt in 1945.

He was president of the USA since 1933 and when he was elected he had a blood pressure (BP) of 140/100 mm Hg. His doctor was an otolaryngologist, Dr. Ross McIntyre, but he had little knowledge about cardiovascular disease.

Between 1935 and 1941 the American President's BP rose to 190/105 mm Hg and even so his private doctor considered that it was compatible with his age and that his patient was still healthy[90].

Roosevelt was not diagnosed with cardiovascular disease until 1944, after the intervention of his daughter, Anna Roosevelt, who demanded that her father be seen by a cardiologist, Dr. Howard Bruenn, one of the few existing at the time in the USA.

In his first evaluation, Dr. Bruenn considered his patient to be hypertensive and also already showing heart failure. His therapeutic options were few and he recommended only a digitalis (cardiotonic used for heart failure) and a low sodium diet (to try to control high blood pressure).

On April 12, 1945, with a BP of 300/190 mm Hg, Roosevelt died at the age of 63 due to cerebral hemorrhage.

This episode caused great commotion among the American population, which led Roosevelt's successor, Harry Truman, to sign a decree law providing $ 500,000 to conduct an epidemiological study on heart disease, in addition to creating the *National Heart Institute,* currently known as *National Heart, Lung and Blood Insitute.*

A young doctor, Gilcin Meadors, was assigned the task of writing a proposal for the epidemiological study.

In a work published in 1951, the planning, methodology and objectives of the study were outlined[91].

It was the first long-term epidemiological long-term study carried out in the USA, and currently this type of study is called a cohort study.

For situations like those at the time of Roosevelt's death, where little was known about the causes of cardiovascular disease, this type of research was ideal.

Cohort studies provide the best type of information on the etiology of diseases that are still unclear, although they are expensive and require prolonged follow-up periods, as was the case in the Framingham study.[92].

He initially focused on hypertensive and arteriosclerotic cardiovascular disease, as they are the most important and of which there was little knowledge at the time.

As a working hypothesis, the researchers assumed that these diseases did not have a single cause, such as infectious diseases, but that they were the result of multiple causes.

They also believed that the existing diagnostic tests were inaccurate and inefficient.

Based on these premises, the study had the following design: to randomly select a group of people in a known age range for the development of hypertensive cardiovascular disease and among these people, after clinical and laboratory evaluation, to find a group free of signs of these diseases.

These would be normal people and would be followed over time, until a reasonable number of them came to acquire the diseases.

At that time, a search would be made to find the factors that would have influenced the development of the disease in one group of people and not in another.

The city of Framingham, Massachusetts, was chosen because it had a population of adults considered statistically reasonable for the study and its proximity to Boston, where many cardiologists from *Harvard Medical School* worked and who provided support for the study. of the works.

Initially, we worked with a cohort of 5,209 people, with ages varying from 28 to 62 years old, with women constituting just over half of the group.

The hypotheses with which the researchers initially worked were as follows:

1. Cardiovascular diseases increase with age, occur early and affect mainly male people.
2. People with hypertension develop cardiovascular disease at a higher rate than normotensive people.
3. Elevated blood cholesterol levels are associated with increased cardiovascular disease.
4. Smoking is associated with an increased occurrence of cardiovascular disease.
5. The usual use of alcohol is associated with an increased incidence of cardiovascular disease.
6. The increase in physical activity is associated with a decrease in the development of cardiovascular disease.

7. An increase in thyroid function is associated with a decrease in the development of cardiovascular disease.

8. An increase in the rate of hemoglobin or blood hematocrit is associated with an increased development of cardiovascular disease.

9. An increase in body weight predisposes to cardiovascular disease.

10. There is an increased development of cardiovascular disease in people with diabetes mellitus.

11. There is a higher incidence of cardiovascular disease in people with gout (a disease caused by an increase in uric acid).

At first, the authors tried to work with a multivariable logistic model with seven factors: age, total cholesterol, weight, abnormalities present on the electrocardiogram (ECG), hemoglobin rate, number of cigarettes smoked per day and systolic blood pressure.

The first results of the study were published in 1957 and defined hypertension as a BP greater than or equal to 160/95 mm Hg, well away from the pressure level considered normal today, which is 120/80 mm Hg, for adults.

In addition, they reported a prevalence of coronary heart disease about four times higher among participants who were hypertensive, thus demonstrating a relationship between the two diseases.

Eight years later, in another study, they concluded that stroke was the main consequence of high blood pressure.

Framingham's studies continued with the descendant generations of the initial group, providing more than 50 years of scientific articles publications for more than 50 years, serving to completely change the way of facing cardiovascular diseases and their risk factors.

Before, atherosclerosis was considered a normal and inevitable consequence of aging, as well as hypertension.

It was the studies produced by these researchers that led us to recognize the importance of the main risk factors for cardiovascular diseases, as well as the need to adopt measures to control and modify them, which led to a reduction of almost 60% in mortality due to coronary heart disease in the USA from 1950 to 1999[93].

Currently, the main risk factors recognized for this group of diseases are smoking, high levels of LDL-cholesterol, low levels of HDL-cholesterol, diabetes mellitus, high blood pressure, family history of cardiovascular disease, obesity (mainly central), sedentary lifestyle and alcohol abuse.

In Brazil, only four diseases are responsible for 80% of all deaths among chronic non-communicable diseases: cardiovascular diseases, various types of cancer, chronic respiratory diseases (such as pulmonary emphysema) and diabetes mellitus.

These diseases have common major risk factors, such as smoking, physical inactivity, inadequate diet (such as a diet rich in saturated fats and carbohydrates, leading to obesity, increased LDL-cholesterol and glucose intolerance, a preliminary step for the development of type 2 diabetes mellitus), in addition to alcohol abuse[94].

It is now common sense that smoking causes cancer, but that was not unanimous until recently.

The sharp growth of lung cancer that followed the widespread smoking in the first half of the 20th century suggested some link between smoking and lung cancer, but few studies suggested this link and lacked scientific bases.

Only after 1950 did some studies based on epidemiological studies of the case and control type allow for obtaining more convincing evidence of this link.

Case and control studies are a simpler way to investigate the cause of diseases, particularly in relation to rare diseases.

This methodology includes people with the disease and a control group, consisting of people not affected by the investigated disease.

The researchers collect data on the occurrence of the disease at a certain point in time and on the occurrence of exposures to some common risk factor at some point in the past.

The incidence of the disease in the exposed and unexposed is what will determine whether the factor in question really has any meaning about the origin of the disease.

Among the initial works that gave a more consistent argument about the relationship between smoking and lung cancer can be mentioned that of Richard Doll and Ernst Wynder, both published in 1950[95][96].

In his text, Doll reports that in England and Wales, in just 25 years, that is, from 1922 to 1947, the cases of deaths from lung cancer increased about 15 times.

And that this considerable increase was entirely disproportionate to the population increase corresponding to the period, especially in relation to the older population and which was the most affected by the disease.

His work presented as a hypothesis to try to clarify this increase in cases the increase in smoking, especially that related to the use of cigarettes.

It also sought to verify whether other types of cancer could be linked to smoking, such as carcinoma of the stomach, rectum and colon.

Its control group consisted of patients admitted to the same hospitals, but for other types of diseases other than cancer.

Of the 649 men who participated in the survey, and who had lung cancer, 99.7% were smokers and only **0.3** % did not have this habit. Among the control group, that is, without cancer, **4.2** % were non-smokers, a difference of **14** times.

The study has not yet shown any correlation between smoking and other types of cancer, such as stomach, rectum and colon cancer.

In his work - which is still considered a milestone in the history of research on smoking and lung cancer - Wynder justifies the need for conducting the research due to the fact that until that moment there was a lack of controlled and large-scale studies to be able to prove whether the smoking was actually implicated in the development of bronchogenic carcinoma.

In his conclusion, he stated that among 605 men with lung carcinoma, 96.5% were moderate to severe smokers for many years, compared with only 73.7% of smokers among the control group without cancer.

And even though the occurrence of lung carcinoma in a non-smoking man - at that time smoking occurred mainly among the male population - it was a rare phenomenon, in the order of 2% of cases.

But, despite all the evidence, it was only in 1962, at the recommendation of President John F. Kennedy, that a committee was created to seek to resolve this issue definitively.[97].

This committee, *Surgeon General's Advisory Committee* (SGAC), was made up of two members of the tobacco industry and ten researchers, including an epidemiologist and a statistician.

The committee sought to gather the relevant evidence, considering the data from the following sources for the development of its work: animal experiments, clinical and anatomopathological studies, in addition to epidemiological studies.

Among the epidemiological studies, 29 case and control studies and seven cohort studies were analyzed, comprising what was best at the time in terms of studies with greater weight and scientific evidence.

In 1964 the SGAC concluded that smoking caused lung cancer in men and that data for women, although in smaller numbers, pointed in the same direction.

And he said that smoking is a health risk in the United States of sufficient importance to ensure that appropriate corrective measures are taken.

These measures, which Congress was responsible for, were taken in the following years, such as regulating the use and sale of tobacco products; placing health warnings on cigarette packages; in addition to restricting advertising in the media, especially on radio and television.

Since that time, new measures have been implemented, especially after the discovery of health damage caused by passive smokers[98].

Thus, over the years, several epidemiological evidences were sufficient to conclude that smoking is the cause of several different types of cancer; cardiovascular diseases (such as atherosclerosis, coronary artery disease and stroke); chronic obstructive pulmonary disease (pulmonary emphysema); acute respiratory diseases (such as pneumonia and asthma attacks); reproductive effects such as inhibition of fetal growth (low birth weight); complications of pregnancy, premature birth, decreased pregnancy and sudden infant death syndrome; osteoporosis leading to hip fracture; in addition to a lower general level of health even in the clinical absence of disease.

As it was later revealed, from the publication of its internal reports, the tobacco industry was carefully trying to escape the emerging scientific evidence.

Instead of recognizing the truths of which they were widely aware, they deliberately tried to falsely reassure the public, especially smokers, that the question of whether smoking actually caused harm to health was still a controversial issue. [99].

However, from the publication of the SGAC report in 1964, the prevalence of smokers in the USA fell from 42% in 1965 to 19% in 2010, that is, a decrease of 55%.

It is estimated that, during this period, this decrease was able to prevent the death of eight million Americans and that they would be caused by the habit of smoking.

Acquired Immunodeficiency Syndrome (AIDS or AIDS)

Like AIDS, syphilis was - from the Middle Ages until the discovery of penicillin - an endemic disease that caused millions of deaths and brought panic to society. Unknown to their cause, syphilitics came to be as discriminated against as lepers, and many times one disease was confused with the other.

When it was realized that it was through sexual contact that the disease was transmitted, prostitutes began to suffer strong persecution, as shown by this preaching, made by one of the greatest anatomists of the time, the French Sylvius, in 1567:

"He learns to hate prostitutes' debauchery more than dogs and snakes. He hates her impudent look, her tempting gestures, her seductive conversations, the sly smile on her lips, her breasts raised to corruption".

As in the late twentieth century - when AIDS generated prejudices and even harassment of so-called risk groups (homosexuals, bisexuals, hemophiliacs, etc.) - at the beginning of the epidemic, syphilis also generated the same feelings of intolerance and irrationality.

The risk of contagion and, as a consequence, of dying from the disease, triggered a new morality, previously quite liberal, and the same happened with AIDS, at least until the emergence of new drugs more effective than the first launched on the market., AZT.

Unlike syphilis - whose causative agent, the bacterium Treponema pallidum, was only discovered in 1905, by Fritz Schaudin, 500 years after its arrival in Europe - the HIV virus, which causes AIDS, was identified in a few years by Montagnier, of the Pasteur Institute, in 1983.

Today, AIDS remains a major public health problem, but especially for underdeveloped countries, such as those in central Africa. Due to the high cost of treating AIDS patients, as it is a chronic disease that can lead to opportunistic infections, some of them requiring hospitalization, the final cost is usually so high that it has had very serious repercussions for the economy of these countries.

The projection of the World Health Organization was that, until the year 2000, there will be about 30 million HIV carriers in the world, with 10 million AIDS cases, 90% of them in underdeveloped countries.

According to another statistic, presented at the XI International AIDS Conference, held in 1996, in Vancouver, Canada, there would be, worldwide, 22 million adults and children with HIV, 94% of them in developing countries.

In Brazil, according to the Ministry of Health, 506 thousand AIDS cases were reported until June 2008, with 205 thousand deaths.

Until 1995 the fatality rate was 9.7 deaths per 100 thousand inhabitants. With the introduction of the policy of universal access to antiretroviral treatment, there was a gradual decrease in mortality, with stabilization at 6.3 deaths per 100 thousand inhabitants, starting in the year 2000.

It is also important to highlight the frequent association of tuberculosis with AIDS, with around 20% to 30% of AIDS cases being reported along with mycobacteriosis, especially among the population with a lower level of education and income.

Studies also show that co-infection with Koch's bacillus and HIV can increase the risk of developing tuberculosis by up to 25 times, which, in turn, significantly contributes to increase AIDS lethality.

Eurico de Aguiar

Dengue

Currently, dengue is the most important viral disease transmitted by mosquitoes that affects humans. Its global distribution is comparable to that of malaria.

The disease is endemic in Africa, the Americas and parts of the Middle East, Asia and the Western Pacific.

The infection is transmitted by Aedes aegypti, a vector of daytime habits. The mosquito is originally from Africa, but has spread to tropical regions of the planet over the past two centuries through international trade. Well adapted to the urban environment, it grows in areas where water is stored or where it can accumulate, such as collections of standing water, bottles, vases, pots, plastic containers and tires. The highest incidence of the disease coincides with the rainy season, which in our country is highest between the months of January to May.

Recent work has shown that the strategy of combating the adult form of the mosquito by spraying with insecticide is no longer the best way to combat the disease. Several populations of the mosquito are resistant to organophosphate insecticides.

The combat to the transmitter must be done, as a priority, to prevent its multiplication from the beginning. For this, the support of the population is essential, as well as the work performed by the teams of the Family Health Program.

The frequency of dengue and its more severe complications, such as the hemorrhagic form and shock syndrome, has grown markedly since the 1980s.

Dengue is a viral disease caused by one of four serotypes of the genus Flavivirus. Infection by one of the serotypes does not provide protection for any other.

As for the clinical form, the disease can range from a non-specific viral syndrome to the most severe forms.

Dengue hemorrhagic fever is a condition with a high risk of death, characterized by increased capillary permeability that can lead to hypovolemic shock and then to death. The hemorrhagic form is detected, laboratorially, by a considerable drop in the blood platelet count.

For the development of severe forms of infection, risk factors are the type of strain and serotype of the virus, as well as age, immunity status, genetic predisposition of the patient and previous contact with another serotype previously.

The type 2 and type 3 dengue epidemic, which mainly affected Rio de Janeiro, produced over 85 thousand cases throughout Brazil, in the first three months of 2008, with more than 400 cases of hemorrhagic form, in addition to dozens of deaths.

There is no specific treatment for dengue virus infection, that is, the treatment is only symptomatic and supportive, especially in cases of suspected severe forms, such as rehydration and control of the hemorrhagic condition.

Covid-19

Eurico de Aguiar

In December 2019, in Wuhan, China, a new beta coronavirus, similar to the SARS agent and the MERS, causing cases of severe acute respiratory syndrome, the call Covid-19.

The new virus, responsible for the disease and called SARS - CoV- 2, was probably transmitted by bats, a mammal responsible for several other zoonoses, such as the one caused by Ebola.

Unlike the rest of the world, by the end of March the disease began to be controlled in China, after the implementation of severe measures of containment and control.

The Covid-19 pandemic is considered an unprecedented global crisis. Halfway September 2020 were recorded, worldwide, 22 million cases and 930,000 deaths (4.2% of the total). In Brazil, until the second half of November 2020, there were nearly 6 million infections and 166 thousand deaths, second highest incidence of cases and of deaths, only less of that what happened in the US.

At least 186 countries have implemented some type of movement restriction to decrease the transmission of the disease, and these restrictions led to a "lockdown" in 82 countries.

World Bank projections consider this to be the biggest economic recession since World War II, with millions of people losing their jobs and their source of income, and, as a result, substantially raising the levels of poverty and misery in several countries.

The conditions most prevalent for development of the disease is will the diabetes to obesity (BMI> or = 30), the c ancer and the cardiovascular diseases, in addition to DOS elderly and smokers, with its comorbidad more prevalents.

The incubation period of the disease usually varies between one and two weeks, and the symptoms of the disease are usually those related to a respiratory virus infection, such as fever, cough, sore throat and respiratory distress. Some patients may have other symptoms, such as myalgia, fatigue, changes in taste and smell. Still others may have gastrointestinal symptoms, such as diarrhea, vomiting and abdominal pain.

The weigh most cases be considered as mild or moderate (or even asymptomatic), portions of affected patients (around 5%) see the present severe, with organ failure, especially respiratory failure, leading to death in a significant proportion.

The most accurate test for diagnosing the disease is RT-PCR (polymerase chain reaction - reverse transcriptase), based on the collection of a sample of nasal or oropharyngeal secretion.

The most frequent radiological finding, among severe cases, is bilateral pulmonary opacity, and computed tomography is more sensitive than the common radiological exam.

The most severe cases usually have the following characteristics:

- Respiratory rate > or = 30 / minute.

- Oxygen saturation < or = 93%.

- Development of respiratory failure requiring ventilatory assistance.

- Shock occurs.

- Need for hospitalization and intensive care unit, monitoring and treatment due to complications with organ failure.

Among severe cases no antiviral treatment was effective, with the best performance drugs so far are those who sought to combat excessive inflammatory reaction of the organism - "cytokine storm" - as dexametazone , and anticoagulants to prevent phenomena thrombotic, common in severe cases.

The humoral immunity response to SARS-CoV-2 is mediated mainly by antibodies directed to the glycoproteins on the viral surface, especially the glycoprotein S ("spike"). These antibodies neutralize infection in human cells and tissues that express the angiotensin-converting enzyme (ACE2), through which the virus penetrates cells to initiate the infection process.

Until August 2020, several types of vaccines were already in phase 3 of clinical trials, involving thousands of participants, such as that of AstraZeneca (United Kingdom), that of Pfizer, Johnson & Johnson and Sinovac Biotech (China).

It is likely that in the first half of 2021, effective vaccines will be available to prevent this disease caused by the new coronavirus.

Relics of the art of cure

In every issue related to the disease, credulity remains a permanent fact, without the influence of civilization or education. Sir William Osler

Contraceptive prescription (Egypt 2200 BC)

Acacia tips well crushed, together with honey and dates, in a wad of fibers, to be introduced deep into the belly.

Prescription for the sex of the child (Egypt 2200 BC)

Fill two bags, made of fabrics, with grains of wheat

and barley. The pregnant woman should water the bags with her urine every day. If the grains in one of the bags start to sprout, she will give birth. If barley sprouts, a girl will be born. If wheat sprouts, a boy will be born. If neither wheat nor barley sprouts, there will be no birth.

Prescription against cold (Egypt, 1500 a. C.)

"Deflux, cold, son of the cold that breaks bones, destroys the skull, so that the seven openings in the heads of Ra's subjects, who now turn to Thot in prayers. See that I brought the medicine against you. Milk from who gave birth to a boy, latex with a pleasant smell that keeps you away. Go to the land, rot, rot four times".

Plants used by traditional Chinese medicine

Yuzhizi: extracted from the dry, ripe fruit of the Akebia quinata plant. Its active principle is saponin. It has a diuretic and anti-inflammatory action.

Zexie: extracted from the dry root of Alisma orientalis. Its active ingredient is alisol. Diuretic action, treatment of hypercholesterolemia and inhibition of platelet aggregation (less chance of thrombosis and stroke).

Garlic: extracted from the plant Allium satimm, also widely used by the Egyptians. Its active ingredient is allicin. Action in the treatment of infectious diseases (antibacterial, antifungal and antiviral). Antilipemic, especially because it leads to a decrease in bad cholesterol (LDL and VLDL cholesterol). It increases the fibrinolytic activity of the blood and inhibits platelet aggregation. It improves the level of glucose tolerance, collaborating to control diabetes.

Anemone: extracted from the plant Anemona raddeana. Its active ingredients are saponins. Anti-rheumatic and anti-inflammatory action (anti-riflebite).

Angelica: extracted from the plant of the same name. Its active ingredient is angelicin. Analgesic, antipyretic, antirheumatic action and for the treatment of uterine hemorrhages.

Anisodus: extracted from the Chinese plant Anisodus tanguticus. Its active principle is an alkaloid called anisodamine / anisodine. Antispasmodic action at the level of arterioles, improving microcirculation. It also has antiasthmatic action, by inhibiting the contraction of the bronchi, when provoked by the action of histamine, as in allergies.

Artemisia: extracted from the bud and leaves of Artemisia annua. Its active ingredient is artemisinin. It has a potent antimalarial action against several species of Plasmodium. In a study of more than two thousand patients with malaria, all were cured with the use of artemisinin, in addition to being effective in treating malaria by chloroquine-resistant Plasmodium falciparum.

Yadanzi: extracted from the ripe fruit of the Brucea gavanica plant. Its active principle is quassinoids. It used to be used as an antimalarial drug, today it is used to treat leukemias.

Cephalotaxus: extracted from eight species of the Cephalotaxus plant. Its active ingredients are alkaloids such as taxol and cephalotaxin. Employed in tumor chemotherapy (cancer).

Duzhong: extracted from the stem of the Eucommia ulmoides plant. Its active principle is aucubine. Antihypertensive action on the smooth muscles of the arterioles, causing vasodilation.

Baigno: extracted from the mature seeds, roots and leaves of the Ginkgo biloba plant. Its active ingredients are gincolidos and phenols. Antimicrobial action given by phenols, improvement of brain activity in the elderly and peripheral vascular irrigation, through scavenger.

Ginseng: extracted from the dry root of the Panax ginseng plant. Its active ingredients are saponins. Very varied action, including cardiovascular effects, on the nervous system, immunity, antitumor and antidiabetic activity. On the cardiovascular system its action is to increase the heart rate and decrease blood pressure. Decreases levels of bad blood cholesterol and triglycerides. Increases levels of good cholesterol (HDL). It has antidiabetic action by decreasing blood glucose levels and increasing glycogen formation in the liver.

Plants used by the Mesopotamians (700 BC)

They knew several medicinal plants such as poppy (source of opium), mandrake, henbane, bay leaf, myrrh, incense, saffron, thyme, cumin, juniper, garlic and onion. The most important, however, was the belladonna, Atropa belladona. Its most important chemical component is atropine, an alkaloid that works by inhibiting the parasympathetic nervous system and that can lead to death if administered in excessive doses.

Hemp, Cannabis sativa, has been used since ancient times in China, India and Mesopotamia. It was used against pain, in cases of bronchitis, bladder diseases, rheumatism and insomnia. It was also used in divination and exorcism.

Prescription against cough (Mesopotamia, 700 BC)

Break up euphorbia[100] in pure beer, honey and refined olive oil. Make the patient swallow the liquid at once. Then have cold beer and honey. Then induce vomiting with the aid of a feather. Then the patient should eat pastries with cream and honey, and drink sweet wine.

Recipe for eliminating kidney stones (Mesopotamia, 700 BC)

Reduce the size of the stones with turpentine oil and powdered eggshells, especially ostrich egg.

Treatment of pneumonia (Mesopotamia 700 BC)

Make hot linseed poultices, combining with wrapping in cloths, which should be dipped repeatedly in hot water or in a fennel tea.

On teaching surgery (India 400 BC)

"The master should make sure that his student learns surgical practice, even if he has already studied the different parts of general medical science. As much as he has read, the student is incompetent as a surgeon, if he does not master the surgical practice. He who knows only his books will be disoriented and frightened when faced with the real disease, like a coward on the battlefield ".

On medical ethics (India 400 BC)

"You dedicate yourself entirely to helping the patient, even with the loss of your own life. Never harm the patient, not even in thought. Strive constantly to improve your knowledge. Do not treat your wife except in the presence of your husband. The doctor must observe all the rules of good dress and good behavior. When you are with a patient, you should not be concerned with words or thoughts of any other subject than the one who suffers. Outside the patient's home he will not be able to talk about the events in that home. You will not be able to talk to the patient about the possibility of his death, when this will harm the patient himself or anyone else. Before the gods you must assume this responsibility. May all the gods assist you when you do so. Otherwise, they are against you. To that students say: so be it ".

On the nature of things (Tito Lucrécio Caro, 59 a. C.)

"Death, in itself, is not terrible; only our fears of the beyond make it so. But the beyond does not exist. Hell is here, in the suffering that arises from ignorance, passion, bellicose and greed; and heaven is here, in the serene temples of wisdom ".

On how to deal with frustrations (Seneca, 65 AD)

We better endure the frustrations for which we prepare and that we understand, and we are affected mainly by those that we least expect and that we cannot understand.

When we rationally face the consequences of an unfulfilled desire, we will have a great chance of realizing that the issues involved tend to be much more modest than the anxieties they generated.

Philosophy must seek to harmonize us with the perception of reality and thus save us, if not from frustration itself, at least from the pernicious emotions that usually accompany it, such as anger or even fits of fury or crises of sadness.

Wisdom is in correctly distinguishing situations in which we are free to shape reality according to our desires, from those in which we are obliged to accept what we cannot change with tranquility and spirit

unarmed.

Ash Wednesday sermon (Father Antônio Vieira, 17th century)

" To die for many years and live many years is not the same thing. Ordinarily men die many years and live a few.
Also the bodies under the earth, also the bones in the graves accompany the courses of time and no one will say it lived.
The our actions are our days; for them the years are counted, for them life is measured: while we work rationally, we live;

the other time we last ".

Recipe for aromatic fumigation (England, 1655)

Take mastic and frankincense, one ounce each, cider pills, pennyroyal roots, dried herbs and cloves, and three drachmas from each. Do everything in a coarse powder and boil over a low heat, in a pot scented with lavender water and white wine.

Recommendations for the preservation of health (Escola de Salerno, 18th century)

Breathe a serene, bright air of purity,

Of which no exhalation obscures clarity;

Avoid infectious odors and harmful vapors,

That rise from the sewers and plague the atmosphere.

Do you want to prolong the success of your pleasures?

Avoid excess addiction and the table.

If evil is insistent, it is up to art to react:

More than curing evil, art must prevent.

Air, rest and sleep, pleasure and food,

They preserve the health of man, if tasted with measure.

Abuse turns this innocent good into poison,

Destroying the body and muddling the mind.

Recipes against sadness (Portugal, 1759)

"Plínio said that good foods banish sadness and calm passions; and I say that the good company of the table is still more effective than the same delicacies that are eaten in it".

"If Cicero called the death of man idleness, also with the Catholic maxim he can call literary employment life, because the recreation of books is a Christian policy for the conformity of evils, and to tolerate them with a cheerful and heroic face to be happy, without depending on fortune".

The difference between the true and the false doctor (England, 1840)

The false presents the same remedy in all diseases, although they may differ widely in their symptoms and character, whereas the true examines, in the spirit of philosophical analysis, all the peculiarities existing in his patient, as well as his disagreement. Hence it adapts with judicious discretion and with a correct judgment of its medicinal agents, in such a way that it can be the best calculated to control and correct your patient's illness.

Remedy for monthly evacuation (Brazil, 1843)

Take a cotton seed stick, infuse it in boiling water, for 20 minutes, with enough volume for a cup, and it should be taken in the morning, on an empty stomach. Being taken six days before the monthly evacuation should appear.

The wisdom of life (Arthur Schopenhauer, 1851)

"Men intend a thousand times more to become rich than to acquire culture, although it is certain that what a man is contributes much more to his happiness than what he has".

Truth and research (Claude Bernard, 1865)

"When I'm in my laboratory, I start by closing the door on materialism and spiritualism; I observe only the facts, and I try only to find the conditions under which life manifests itself."

"When you encounter a fact that is opposed to an established theory, you must adhere to the facts and abandon the theory, even if it is supported by great authorities and usually adopted."

On experimental science (Louis Pasteur, 1884)

"The will is powerful, while action and work generally follow the will and work is almost always accompanied by success. These three things, will, work and success, fill human existence. The will opens the doors to success brilliantly and happily; work goes through these doors and at the end of the journey, success comes to crown our efforts. And then, if your determination is firm, your task will be how it can be done, if you have already started it; and you will have to walk ahead if you want to complete it.

The cultivation of science, in its maximum expression, is perhaps even more necessary for a nation's moral condition than for its material prosperity.

Great discoveries, such as the manifestations of thought in

art, science and letters, and in a word the disinterested exercise of the mind in each direction and in the instruction centers from which they radiate, introduce society, as a whole, into the philosophical spirit and scientific, in the spirit of discernment that submits everything to severe reasoning, condemns ignorance and discards error and prejudice. "They raise the intellectual level and the moral sense, and through them the divine idea itself is disseminated and intensified".

Beyond good and evil (Nietzsche, 1886)

"The greatest successes and the greatest ideas (the greatest ideas are the greatest successes) are understood very late: contemporary generations do not live them, although they live alongside them. It happens in life as in the realm of the stars. The light from the most distant stars comes to us late, and yet, man denies that such stars exist. How many centuries does a spirit need to be understood? This too is a measure, a hierarchy is also created, as well as among spirits as well as stars.

How to Treat Nerve Attacks (France, 1909)

The attack of nerves, also called nervous breakdown or hysterical crisis, is specific to some nervous or emotional women or young people. It can also occur in men, but more rarely.

The crisis is sometimes announced in advance of several hours, or even days, through yawns, tears or laughter for no reason, or by a sensation of the presence of a ball rising from the abdomen or chest to the neck.

The crisis explodes as a result of emotion, annoyance or even for no apparent reason, especially during the menstrual period.

Open the windows and give the patient air, remove his clothes, lay him on a sofa or on a bed. Remove all unnecessary people around you. If you are a young woman, leave only your mother. If you are a lady, just leave your husband by your side.

Throw cold water on your face. If the crisis is severe, those who attend can try to compress, with both hands, strongly, on the lower abdomen, in the region of the ovaries, especially on the left side.

Do not give salts, or strong odors, vinegars, or anything else that could excite the patient and prolong the crisis. But you can, with a handkerchief, make her inhale a little ether or cologne.

The attacks end with abundant tears or a little delirium. If they recur, a doctor should be consulted who will seek to find the primary reasons for these attacks and indicate the appropriate treatment to be followed.

How to prevent baldness (France, 1911)

Daily massage the scalp with the following solution: Ammonia - 4 gr .; Turpentine essence - 13 gr.e Camphorated alcohol - 83 ml.

How to treat diabetes (France, 1911)

Therapeutic indications:

Body hygiene - Warm baths, twice a week, for 20 minutes, accompanied by gentle rubbing with a sponge.

Food hygiene - Restriction of sugar, which should be replaced by glycerin or saccharin. Restrict fruits, except peaches, apricots, apples, raspberries and melons, all in small quantities. Restrict flour. Vegetables are allowed, as well as fats, butter, oil, eggs and cheese. Small amount of bread. Meat and fish are also allowed. Pasta should be restricted. Alcohol, none.

How to treat epilepsy (France, 1911)

For crisis prevention, prepare a chloral hydrate solution, which should be given up to three times every 24 hours, when the attacks are repeated at short intervals.

Method of preparation of the solution: Chloral hydrate - 2 gr.; Potassium bromide - 2 gr.; Egg yolk - 01. Water - 150 ml.

Chloroform can also be used (via the nasal route), but its action is more uncertain, the same with ether and ethyl bromide. The patient should be kept in a dimly lit room, where he will be prohibited from speaking or moving.

How to treat insomnia (France, 1911)

At dusk, before the last meal, take a bath with salts, lasting 45 minutes, at a temperature of 36/37 ºC.

Then, have a light meal, without alcohol or coffee. Go to bed after two and a half hours after the meal is finished.

Psychotherapy (France, 1922)

Psychotherapy is a real science of which we will give only a few indications here. Just remember that:

Every doctor who enjoys the trust of a patient performs a favorable action on him, which contributes strongly to the therapeutic success.

Although useful at all times and in all places, this action is particularly indispensable and precious when trying to treat a nervous or mental illness.

In many cases, it is essential that this psychotherapy has its full effect of isolating the patient, of withdrawing him from the family environment from which the poor treatment worsens most of the pathological manifestations.

This psychotherapy, especially valid in so-called functional disorders of the nervous system, is far from being ineffective when you have an organic disease.

It needs a lot of consistency on the part of the doctor, security, psychological talent and in-depth knowledge of the case to be treated.

Hysteria (France, 1922)

Prevention:

Raise children in a convenient way, save them violent emotions, develop their reason and intelligence above all. If you are dealing with people with neuropathic activity, send them to live in the countryside and see to it that they do not see a hysterical attack.

Treatment:

1st Psychotherapeutic methods - isolation is by far the best way to treat hysteria. Some people are cured just by thinking about entering a nursing home. For others, remember that isolation must be absolute. That there are frequent visits by the doctor, who must care and make efforts on an ongoing basis and reducing the severity until the patient is cured.

2nd Physical methods - electricity acts, above all, by suggestion. So, it is one of the most precious medications, when it is well managed. As for hydrotherapy, if we apply it, preferably use warm showers.

Breastfeeding the newborn (Germany, 1922)

The child should not receive any food on the first day after delivery. The mother needs to rest, and, in addition, the newborn, in general, does not show signs of hunger. If you feel uncomfortable, you can simply give a few small spoons of thin tea, sweetened with a little sugar, to which is added a pinch of salt.

On the second day (24 hours after delivery), the child will be taken to the breast for the first time. For this, the mother, lying down, turns to the son placed beside her. Then, with the nipple pinned by it between the index and middle fingers, it will be introduced into the child's mouth in such a way that it does not suck only the nipple, but is able to trap the entire aureolar vestibule between the jaw and jaw. However, be careful to let the child's nose free, which should not stick to the chest, due to the risk of suffocation.

On the first day, breastfeeding begins, taking the infant to the breast more or less three times. The next day, four times, and thereafter five times, with regular four-hour breaks, keeping an eight-hour break during the night. If the child is uneasy during the night, a little tea can be given in the first few weeks, until they get used to the big night break.

Many children, when the secretion is abundant, are content with four feedings a day. The habit of feeding at the right time means that the infant does not require food during breaks. But, when you occasionally show hunger just before the scheduled time, or when you are asleep exceeds the prescribed time for breastfeeding, there is no inconvenience in departing a little from this regime.

The time for each feeding should last approximately 20 minutes. When the child sucks badly, or for some reason finds it difficult to breastfeed, the time can be increased to thirty minutes during the first week of life.

After three days of delivery, the nursing mother should sit on the bed to breastfeed her child.

Exclusive breastfeeding of the child should go until the sixth month of life. Thereafter, one of the feedings should be replaced by a soup (made with broth or boiled vegetables), to which is added a little flour (barley, etc.), until it acquires the consistency of soft pirão, do which is given to the child from 150 to 200 grams. Thus, it is gradually passed to artificial feeding, until weaning occurs around the ninth month or until the first year of life.

How to treat obesity (France, 1922)

Every obese person who wants to lose weight must have patience and willpower, eat alone or in an appropriate sanatorium, and weigh themselves regularly each week.

All the desired regimes rest on the same principle: reducing the mass of food and choosing its quality.

Foods to avoid: fatty meats, sauces, butter, cold cuts, puree, sweets and chocolates.

Drinks to avoid: beer, liquors, alcohol, wine, champagne and cider.

Examples of dietary regimens:

1. For the big obese - bed rest.

First week: 3 to 4 liters of milk per day, and one or two eggs.

Second week: 3 liters of milk, and one egg a day.

Third week: 3 liters of milk per day. The patient will rise.

Fourth week: 2 liters of milk per day. Some exercises, like walking.

2. For the average obese.

Breakfast: cup of warm tea, with a little lemon juice.

Lunch: grilled steak, salad with a little oil, vinegar and lemon juice. Spinach or chicory. A fruit. A piece of grilled bread.

Dinner: chicken or bird or game, without sauce and in small quantities. Salad. A fruit. A piece of grilled bread.

Refrain from beer, liquors, sugar, cakes, and put too little salt in food. Water at will.

Complement to the diet, for people without other health problems: physical exercises (long walks, swimming, skating, etc.) practiced following a methodical script. Hot baths, steam baths and massages.

Obese people with cardiac complications: do not proceed with a weight loss cure unless with extreme caution.

The defense of homeopathy (France, 1922)

"Homeopathy, which we could more accurately call homeotherapy, is a therapeutic method almost unknown to modern doctors. She is, however, as old as the world. Hippocrates defined the principle as one of the foundations of medicine. She was always employed. Paracelsus, Van Helmont, Sthal founded their therapy on her, but on the day that she was erected in doctrine by Samuel Hahnemann it seems that she came to be seen as an excommunicated young heretic. It is necessary, at least, to know what it is about:

The principle of homeopathy is this: "the like are healed by the like". When we read the ancient authors, we realized that this idea almost always governed their therapy, and that they resorted to the law that we can enunciate: similia similibus curantur.

Definitely, the homeopath, in front of a patient, analyzes him at length, looks for all the symptoms that he presents and administers the medicine that will restore his health. This principle having been put, a consequence necessarily follows from it. It is necessary to know the action on the healthy man of the remedies applied to him. Hahnemann, and later his disciples, systematically studied (about themselves and their students) a considerable amount of substances, carefully writing down their effects, sensations, psychic and physical changes, and in this way edited an immense work that they called "pure medical matter".

A second consequence of the similarity law was the lowering of doses. It was not a preconceived idea. Hahnemann used, at first, very strong doses of medicine, to the point that his compatriots called him dangerous. Little by little, he realized that these doses started, before curing, by exaggerating the morbid state, which is easily conceived. Then he noticed that the lower doses not only did not aggravate, but they healed better and faster.

More and more attenuating the doses, he reached infinitesimal doses, daily used since then by his followers, although homeopathy is no longer conceived as separable from the use of infinitesimal doses.

In short, homeopathy is a therapeutic method that treats diseases by the remedies that produce on man the same symptoms presented by the patient. Corollary is the need to study the effects produced by these remedies on healthy men and the use of infinitesimal doses.

How to prevent headache and migraine (France, 1925)

a) Avoid brain fatigue, physical inactivity, immobility, confinement; live in a well-ventilated environment, and exercise regularly.

b) Make light meals, preferably vegetarian: eggs, creams, soups, purees, fruits, salads and breads. Drink plenty of fluids. Avoid foods that contain chocolate.

c) Avoid constipation by using a laxative regime, using washes and suppositories. Use cold compresses on the belly.

d) Act on the skin by means of hot baths: keep the water, above the shoulders, at a temperature of 38 to 40ºC, every morning.

On the choice of medicine (Sigmund Freud, 1935)

"Although we lived in very limited circumstances, my father insisted that, in choosing a profession, I should follow my own inclinations. Neither at that time, nor, indeed, for the rest of my life, did I feel any special predilection for a medical career-. I was driven more by a kind of curiosity, which was, however, directed more towards human concerns than towards natural objects, nor had I recognized the importance of observation as one of the best ways to be gratified. At the same time, Darwin's theories, then of great interest, attracted me strongly, because they extended our hopes for an extraordinary advance in our understanding of the world. And listening to Goethe's beautiful essay on nature, read aloud at a conference I attended just before I left school, led me to decide to study medicine ".

On the history of science (George Sarton, 1941)

"The history of science, and in particular the history of medicine, is not simply an account of discoveries. Its purpose is to explain the development of the scientific spirit, the history of man's reactions to the truth, the history of the gradual release of our minds from darkness and prejudice ".

On the complexity of nature (John Barrow, 1994)

"There is a form of chaos that is caused by excessive order; by many laws; for a lot of complexity. Our confidence in the simplicity of Nature can be undeserved. Nature may seem simple to us only because it has revealed very little of its secrets. As we go deeper into the microscopic structure of matter and space-time, we will be able to discover a vein of great complexity created by the simultaneous interaction of a huge number of factors. Such a situation can seem like lawless, like pure chaos ".

On the art of life (Zygmunt Bauman, 2009)

"No matter in which direction you look, reflection on the art of life ultimately leads to the idea of self-determination and self-assertion, and the willpower that facing such an amazing task necessarily requires. Being yourself consists in resolutely rejecting and repelling definitions and identities imposed or implied by others."

Epilogue (About the present and the future)

We need history, but not as idlers who stroll in the garden of science need it. Advantages and disadvantages of history for life
Friedrich Nietzche

      The growing scientific and technological development currently applied to the diagnosis and treatment of various types of diseases - and, mainly, to chronic-degenerative diseases (including terminal diseases) - has led to an uncontrollable increase in the costs of medical and hospital assistance throughout the world, including in developed countries.

In regions where these resources are scarce, such as in Brazil, the model based heavily on curative medicine produces great distortions and terrible dilemmas.

At the same time that the media praises the great advances of a science increasingly supported by an expensive and complex technology, increasingly scarce resources have to be managed to face an immense challenge.

How to serve the most needy populations, subject, even today, to the lack of basic sanitation, nutritional deficiencies of all kinds, exposure to various types of endemic diseases, limited access to an efficient public system, with a lack of decent housing, without access to information, exposed daily to various types of physical and psychological violence, without access to leisure and without professional training that allows you to earn a decent income?

The current model, which favors treatment, generates considerable consumption of public money, in addition to transforming the State into a mere transfer of resources from the public sector to the private sector, to the detriment of the real interests of the vast majority of the population.

This model presents as a manifestation of its bankruptcy the non-correlation between the increase in health spending and infant mortality and life expectancy at birth[101]. Access to medical care tends to vary inversely with the needs of the population and in the relative distribution among different social groups, according to some health indicators.

In the USA, the world's richest country, millions of people are not served by any health system, especially portions of the population made up of poor and black people.

In Brazil, until 1990, the poorest regions, such as the North and Northeast, received only 21% of the resources transferred by the Ministry of Health for outpatient care, while only the South and Southeast, wealthier regions, received the majority, or 72 % of resources[102].

Another relevant issue concerns the government's real spending on health. Studies carried out by the Federal Council of Medicine show that from 2001 to 2013 80.5 billion reais were authorized for investments by the Ministry of Health, but that only 33 billion were actually spent, that is, only 41% of the estimated budget[103].

We still suffer from the culture of hospitalization, in addition to the fact that universities continue to insist on training doctors with strong individualist appeal. They are only prepared to work in hospitals with strong technological support, away from more suitable scenarios for teaching and learning. Community teaching could be an alternative, where there are several opportunities to make student learning much more enriched, while not being repetitive in relation to what is taught in schools and university hospitals.

As an example of these activities, participation in immunization programs, in epidemiological surveys, in the active search of patients with chronic-degenerative diseases (diabetes, hypertension, etc.) or infectious diseases (such as leprosy and tuberculosis), in health surveillance can be cited , in health education, in participation in community development programs, in public schools and in various other areas and activities of social interest.

On the other hand, the medical curriculum has always been characterized by the lack of disciplines in the area of humanities, limiting the humanistic content of formal medical education to isolated topics from related disciplines, such as Medical Ethics and Medical Psychology. This is a mistake, as for those who consider medicine the meeting point of the biological sciences and the human sciences. As a result, the doctor's training is incomplete without humanistic training.

Some colleges in the country have been concerned with these issues and have tried to give the profile of the doctor to be graduated some characteristics that meet these needs. For these faculties, new doctors must, in addition to excellent technical training, have the following skills:

- Practice medicine with an ethical and humanistic attitude towards the patient, family and community.
- Have a social view of the doctor's role.
- Knowing how to work in a multidisciplinary team, relating to other members on an ethical basis.
- Inform and educate their patients, families and community about health promotion, in addition to the prevention, treatment and rehabilitation of diseases, using appropriate communication techniques.
- To be stimulated and qualified for the practice of permanent education, especially for self-learning, a consequence of the need for constant updating, caused by the growing and continuous mass of new information in the health area.

Another issue is the lack of terminal illness at the medical school, causing the residency becomes essential to professional training, which helps to raise the training of specialists rather than general practitioners, as would be more appropriate to meet the greater needs of poorest populations in the country.

In addition, the medical residency - as a general rule - lacks both curriculum guidelines and specific guidelines, that is, the definition of competencies and skills that guide adequate training in each specialty, not to mention the fact that there is no satisfactory regulation and inspection of medical residency courses in our country.

On the other hand, most colleges are not contributing to the

placement in the labor market of professionals adapted to the new demands and challenges demanded by the health problems that will be prevalent in the 21st century.

In this century, psychiatric diseases (mainly anxiety and depression), smoking-related diseases and sexually transmitted diseases (linked to unsafe sex) are expected to increase, in addition to the pathologies associated with them.

Urban violence (with its consequences in terms of public health) and care for the elderly will also increase in importance.

The United Nations considers the period from 1975 to 2025 as the *Age of Aging*, with the decline in birth - motivated mainly by the adoption of better contraceptive practices - and mortality due to the improvement of health technologies being considered as the main responsible for this. , more efficient control of infectious diseases and improvement of sanitary conditions in general.

Thus, health practices will shift from acute illnesses, in young people, to chronic illnesses, in the elderly, a group of people who are characterized by, over time, being less autonomous and more vulnerable.

Attention to families will play an increasingly important role, as will home care. As a result, new organizational structures are expected to emerge in response to new demands, with a focus on disease prevention and health promotion.

The pandemic, caused by the new coronavirus, showed in a very significant way, the importance of being permanently alert to the appearance of new zoonosis. Forest areas are reservatories of several unknown microorganisms, especially viruses. As we enter in these areas - such as through burning, deforestation, mining, etc. - we are subject to having similar problems in the future. Nothing we do against nature goes unpunished. In one way or another, soon or later, mankind will pay the price for the lack of responsibility, greed and selfishness of some.

And the State will still need to invest more in the construction of basic sanitation networks and in improving the quality of the water that is offered to the population. And also in garbage collection and treatment systems, in immunization (including greater diversification of available vaccines), in the construction of rainwater drainage networks and in combating the vectors of the main infectious and parasitic diseases.

We cannot yet forget education, which, in our country, when elitizing knowledge - without providing a basic , free, universal quality education - has prevented the majority of the population from accessing this fundamental right to the construction of citizenship, understood as the concrete expression of the full exercise of democracy, since educating is not only transmitting knowledge, but also forming free citizens and who are builders of a nation project that has as guiding principles values such as freedom, solidarity, peace and development with social justice.

Acnowledgements

To all those who, with their criticisms, reflections and suggestions, contributed to improve this text over time.

To my wife and my whole family for their affection and attention.

To the readers, the reason for this work.

Bibliography

Ackerknecht, EH A short history of medicine. The Ronald Press, Co., New York, 1955.

Adler, MJ, Editor. Hippocrates & Galen, Great books of the western world, 5th Edition, Encyclopaedia Britannica Inc., Chicago, 1994.

Adler, RE Revolutionary doctors; of Hippocrates to the human genome. Ediouro, Rio de Janeiro, 2004.

Alberg, AJ; Shopland, DR and Cummings, KM The 2014 Surgeon General's Report Commemorating the 50th Anniversary of the Report of the Advisory Committee to the US Surgeon General and Updating the Evidence on the Health Consequences of Cigarette Smoking. American Journal of Epidemiology, vol. 179: 403-412, 2014.

Almeida, LD Susceptibility: a new meaning for vulnerability. Revista Bioética; 18 (3): 537-548, 2010.

Almeida, MJ Medical education and health; possibilities for change. Editora UEL, Londrina, 1999.

Andery, MA; Micheletto, N.; Seriously, TMP; Rubano, DR; Moroz, M.; Pereira, ME; Gioia, SC; Gianfaldoni, M.; Savioli, MR and Zanotto, ML To Understand Science, a historical perspective, 9th edition, EDUC, S. Paulo, 2000.

Aranha, MLA History of Education and Pedagogy, 3rd edition, Moderna, S. Paulo, 2006.

Atkinson, DT Magic, myth and medicine, Fawcett Publications, Inc., New York, 1956.

Auber, E. Philosophie de la medicine, Librarie Germer Baillié, Paris, 1865.

Avila-Pires, F. Principles of Medical Ecology, 2nd edition, Editora da UFSC, Florianópolis, 2000.

Barquin, M. History of medicine, his current problem, 5th edition, Francisco Mendez Oteo, editor, Libreria de Medicina, Mexico, DF, 1980.

Barrett, JT Textbook of immunology, 4th edition, The CV Mosby Co., St. Louis, 1983.

Bass, JB, editor. Tuberculosis, North American Medical Clinics, vol. 6, Interlivros, Rio de Janeiro, 1993.

Bauman, Z. The art of life, Zahar, Rio de Janeiro, 2009.

Beckett, W. History of Painting, Editora Ática, S. Paulo, 1997.

Berlingoff, WP and Gouvea, FQ Mathematics through the Times, Editora Blucher, S. Paulo, 2008.

Bernard, C. De la physiologie genérale, Librarie Hachette, Paris, 1872.

_____. La science experimentale, 5éme edition, Librarie JB Bailliére et fils, Paris, 1911.

Bernard, J. Hopes and Wisdom of Medicine, Editora UNESP, S. Paulo, 1997.

Bingham, P.; Verlander, NQ; Cheal, MJ John Snow, William Farr and the 1849 outbreak of cholera that affected London: a reworking of the data highlights the importance of the wáter supply. Public Health, vol. 118: 387-394, 2004.

Boisson, R. History of the doctor. Librarie Larousse, Paris, 1967.

Botelho, JB and Costa, HL Pajé: reconstruction and survival. History, Sciences, Health-Manguinhos, Rio de Janeiro; 13 (4): 927-956, 2001.

Botton, A. The consolations of philosophy, Rocco, Rio de Janeiro, 2001.

Bousquat, A. and Cohn, A. The spatial dimension in health studies: a historical trajectory. History, Sciences, Health - Manguinhos, Rio de Janeiro, Vol.11 (3): 549-568, 2004.

Bouzon, E. The Hammurabi code, Editora Vozes, Petrópolis, 1976.

Braudel, F. Material civilization, economics and capitalism: 15th-18th centuries. Cotian structures, Martins Fontes, S. Paulo, 2005.

_____. Material civilization, economy and capitalism: 15th-18th centuries. The time of the world, Martins Fontes, S. Paulo, 2009.

Brier, B. Infectious diseases in ancient Egypt. Infectious Disease Clinics of North America, 18: 17-27, 2004.

Bonita, R.; Beaglehole, R. and Kjellstr öm, T. Basic epidemiology, 2nd edition, World Health Organization, Livraria Santos Editora, S. Paulo, 2010.

Brody, DE and Brody, AR The seven greatest scientific discoveries in history, Companhia das Letras, S. Paulo, 2001.

Brooks, CM and Cranefield, PF The historical development of physiological thought, The Hafner Publishing Co., New York, 1959.

Bulcão, LG; El-Kareh, AC and Sayd, JD Science and medical education in Brazil (1930-1950). History, Sciences, Health - Manguinhos, Rio de Janeiro, v.14 (2): 469-487, 2007.

Burns, EM History of Western Civilization, 2nd edition, 2 volumes, Editora Globo, Porto Alegre, 1964.

Burns, GW and Bottino, PJ Genética, 6th edition, Guanabara Koogan, Rio de Janeiro, 1991.

Bynum, W. History of Medicine, L&PM Pocket, Porto Alegre, 2011.

_____. A brief history of science. L&PM, Porto Alegre, 2013.

Calder, R. Man and medicine. Boa Leitura Editora, S. Paulo, 1976.

_____. Man and medicine, a thousand years of darkness. Livraria Editora Ltda., S. Paulo, 1976.

Carlini, ELA and Luz, MT Medicina: The question of homeopathy, Ciência Hoje, vol. 7 (39), January / February, 1988.

Castiglioni, A. A history of medicine, 2nd edition, Alfred A. Knopf, New York, 1958.

Cerda, JL and Valdivia, GC John Snow, the cholera epidemic and the birth of clinical epidemiology. Revista Chilena de Infectologia, Vol. 24 (4): 331-334, 2007.

Coelho, EC Imperial professions: medicine, engineering and law in Rio de Janeiro, 1822-1930, Editora Record, S. Paulo, 1999.

Coelho, FRG coordinator. Basic Oncology Course at Hospital AC Camargo, Medsi Editora Ltda., Rio de Janeiro, 1996.

Comby, J. Deux cent soixante medical consultations pour les maladies des enfants, 8th edition, Masson et Cie., Editeurs, Paris, 1925.

_____. Formula du poche pour les maladies des enfants, cinaquiémé édition, Vigot frérés, editeurs, Paris, 1921.

Cowen, DL and Segelman, AB Editors. Antibiotics in historical perspective, Merck & Co. Inc., 1981.

Cruz, O .G. Opera Omnia. Oswaldo Cruz Institute, Rio de Janeiro, 1972.

Damásio, AR Descartes' mistake: emotion, reason and the human brain, Companhia das Letras, S. Paulo, 1996.

Darwin, C. The Origin of Species, by means of natural selection or the preservation of favored races in the struggle for life. Batam Books, New York, 1859.

Davies, K. Deciphering the genome, Companhia das Letras, S. Paulo, 2001.

Dawber, T .; Meadors, G. and Moore Jr., F. Epidemiological approaches to heart disease: The Framingham study. American Journal of Public Health, vol.41: 279-286, 1951.

Del Priore, M. and Venancio, R. A brief history of Brazil, Editora Planeta do Brasil, S. Paulo, 2010.

Desmond, A. & Moore, J. Darwin, the life of a tormented evolutionist, 3rd edition, Geração Editorial, S. Paulo, 2000.

Diepgen, P. History of Medicine, Editorial Labor, Madrid, 1932.

Doll, R. and Hill, AB Smoking and carcinoma of the lung. British Medical Journal, vol.2: 739-748, 1950.

Donini, A. Brief history of religions, Editora Civilização Brasileira, Rio de Janeiro, 1965.

Duncan, BB et al. Chronic noncommunicable diseases in Brazil: priority for coping and research. Revista de Saúde Pública, vol. 46 (Suppl.): 126-134, 2012.

Durant, W. Heroes of History, Ediouro, Rio de Janeiro, 2002.

Entralgo, PL Hippocratic medicine, Ediciones de la revista de occidente, Madrid, 1970.

Etchegoyen, RH Fundamentals of psychoanalytic technique, 2nd edition, Artes Médicas, Porto Alegre, 1989.

Eyler, JM The changing assessments of John Snow's and William Farr's cholera studies. Soz-Präventivmed, vol. 46: 225-232, 2001.

Fac c hi netti, C. et al. In the maze of fountains at the National Hospice for the Alienated. History, Sciences, Health - Manguinhos, Rio de Janeiro, Vol. 17, supl.2, 2010, p.733-768.

Fernandes, AT, chief editor. Hospital Infection and its interactions in the health area, 2 vol., Atheneu, S. Paulo, 2000.

Fernandes, F., coordinator. Habermas, sociology, 3rd edition, Editora Ática, S. Paulo, 1993.

Ferreira Antunes, JL; Nascimento, CB; Nassi, LC Instituto Adolfo Lutz. 100 years of the public health laboratory, Editora Letras & Letras, S. Paulo, 1992.

Feuerwerker, LCM Changes in medical education and medical residency in Brazil, Hucitec / Rede unida, S. Paulo, 1998.

Fonseca, MRF Sources for the history of health sciences in Brazil (1808-1930), History, Sciences, Health - Manguinhos, Rio de Janeiro, vol. 9 (supplement): 275-288, 2002.

Astire formulaire. Vademecum de Médecine Pratique, Librarie du Monde Médical, Paris, 1922.

Foucault, M. History of Madness, Editora Perspectiva, S. Paulo,

Eurico de Aguiar

1972.

Fox, CS et al. Temporal trends in coronay heart disease mortality and sudden cardiac death from 1950 to 1999: the Framingham heart study. Circulation, vol. 110: 522-527, 2004.

Fr iedman, M and Friedland, G. The ten greatest discoveries in medicine, Companhia das Letras, S. Paulo, 2000.

Freud, S. Complete works, 3 volumes, 4th edition, Editorial Biblioteca Nueva, Madrid, 1981.

G. Lemoine et E. Gérard. Formulaire Consultations Médicales et chirurgicales, Vigot Frères, Editeurs, Paris, 1911.

Galesi, VMN and Almeida, MMB Indicators of hospital morbidity and mortality from tuberculosis in the city of São Paulo. Revista Brasileira de Epidemiologia, 10 (1): 48-55, 2007.

Garrison, FH An introduction to the history of medicine, 4th edition, WB Saunders Co., Philadelphia, 1967.

Glasscheib, HS The great secrets of medicine, Livros do Brasil edition, Lisbon, 1961.

Gomes, O .C. History of Medicine in Brazil in the 16th Century, Brazilian Institute of History of Medicine, Rio de Janeiro, 1974.

Gordon, R. The scary history of medicine, 9th edition, Ediouro publications, Rio de Janeiro, 1996.

Goulart, FAA Health, disease and care systems: an overview of the coming decades. Brasília Médica, 2000; 37 (1/2): 46-50.

Work Group - Medical Course, Pedagogical Project. Health Sciences Teaching and Research Foundation, Health Secretariat, Federal District Government, 2001.

Guillebaud, JC The Force of Conviction, Bertrand Brasil, Rio de Janeiro, 2005.

Guillén, DG, Albarracin, A., Arquiola, E., Erill, S., Montiel, L., Peset, JL, and Entralgo, PL Drug History, Glaxo do Brasil, Rio de Janeiro, 1993.

Gunnel, JG Political Theory, Editora Universidade de Brasília, Brasília, 1979.

Guthrie, D. A history of medicine, Thomas Nelson and sons Ltd., London, 1945.

Haggard, HW The doctor in history, Sudamericana Editorial, Buenos Aires, 1962.

Han, E. et al. Lessons learned from using COVID-19n restrictions: a analysis of countries and regions in Asia Pacific and Europe. Lancet 2020; 396: 1525-1534.

Hardman, JG and Limbird, LE, editors. The pharmacological basis of therapeutics, 9th edition, McGraw-Hill, New York, 1996.

Hardy, A. Water and the search for public health in London in the eighteen and nineteen centuries. Medical history, vol. 28 (3): 250-282, 1984.

Hayek, S., translator. Holy Quran. Tangará Expansão Editorial, São Paulo, 1977.

Hegel, GWF Philosophy of History, 2nd edition, Editora Universidade de Brasília, Brasília, 1999.

Heisenberg, W. Physics and Philosophy, 4th edition, Editora Universidade de Brasília, Brasília, 1999.

Herson, B. New Christians and their descendants in Brazilian medicine (1500/1850). EDUSP, S. Paulo, 1996.

Hessen, J. Theory of knowledge, Armenian Amado Editor, Coimbra, 1964.

Hirayama, T. Non-smoking wives of heavy smokers have a high risk of lung cancer. British Medical Journal, vol. 282: 183-185, 1981.

Hobsbawn, E. About History, Editora Schwarcz Ltda., S. Paulo, 1998.

Hohenheim, PT Paracelsus, the key to alchemy. Editora Três, S. Paulo, 1973.

INCA. www.inca.gov.br/estimativa/2014. Accessed on 08/12/2014.

Inzucchi, SE and Sherwin, RS Type 2 diabetes mellitus. In Cecil Medicine, 23rd ed., Elsevier Saunders, Philadelphia, 2008.

Kaplan, HI and Sadock, BJ Compendium of Psychiatry, 7th edition, Artmed, Porto Alegre, 1997.

Kemp, A. and Edler, FC Medical reform in Brazil and the United States: a comparison between two rhetorics. History,

Sciences, Health - Manguinhos, Rio de Janeiro, vol. 11 (3): 569-585, 2004.

Koestler, A. Man and the Universe, IBRASA, S. Paulo, 1989.

Kuhn, T. The structure of scientific revolutions, 3rd edition, Perspectiva, S. Paulo, 1995.

Jacoulet, F. Guide du Médecin Praticien, deuxième édition, Librairie JB Baillière et fils, Paris, 1922.

Kleinschmidt, H. Formulario Pratico de Therapeutica Infantil, 1st Brazilian edition, Pongetti & Cia, Rio de Janeiro, 1925.

Kerr-Pontes, LRS, Oliveira, FAS and Freire, C..M. Tuberculosis associated with AIDS: situation in the Northeast region of Brazil. Revista de Saúde Pública, vol. 31: 323-329, 1997.

Klobentz, GD The threat of pandemic influenza: why today is not 1918, World Medical & Health Policy, vol.1: Iss, Article 9, 2009.

Lai, C. et al. Factors associated with clinical outcomes in patients with Coronavirus Disease 2019 in Guangzhou, China. Journal of Clinical Virology 2020; 133: 1-6.

Leavell, H. and Clark, EG Preventive medicine, Editora MacGraw-Hill do Brasil Ltda., S. Paulo, 1978.

Leonardo, RA History of medical thought, Froben Press, New York, 1946.

Lewis, P. Editor. The History of Medicine, Reed International Books Ltd., New York, 1996.

Lisbon, AMJ The rainbow curriculum. Reflections on medical education, Linha Gráfica Editora, Brasília, 1999.

Lopes, O .C. Medicine in time, Editora da Universidade de S. Paulo, S. Paulo, 1969.

Lopez, A. and Mota, CG História do Brasil - Uma Interpretação, Editora Senac, S. Paulo, 2008.

Lown, B. The lost art of healing. Editora Peirópolis, S. Paulo, 2008.

Lyons, Al.S. and Petrucelli, J., Editores. History of Medicine, Editora Manole Ltda., S. Paulo, 1997.

Machado, CA The role of translation in the transmission of science: the case of Ptolemy's Tetrabiblos. Thesis for obtaining the title of Doctor of Letters at PUC-Rio, Rio de Janeiro, 273 p., 2010.

Macoris, ML, et al. Resistance of Aedes aegypti from the state of São Paulo, Brazil, to organophosphates insecticides. Memories of the Oswaldo Cruz Institute, 98 (5): 703-708, 2003.

Magnoli, D. A drop of blood, Editora Contexto, S. Paulo, 2009.

Mahmood, SS et al. The Framingham heart study and the epidemiology of cardiovascular diseases: a historical perspective. Lancet, vol. 383: 991-1008, 2014.

Mandell, GL, editor. Principles and Practice of infectious diseases, 4th Edition, Churchill Livingstone, New York, 1995.

_____. Principles and Practice of Infectious Diseases, 6th Edition, Churchill Livingstone, New York, 2005.

Marcondes, D. Introduction to the history of philosophy, 12th edition, Zahar, Rio de Janeiro, 2008.

Marcondes, E., Gonçalves, EL Medical Education, Sarvier, S.

Paulo, 1998.

Mastrocolla, LE, Andriolo, A. and Carvalhaes Neto, N. 1st Meeting of Laboratory Medicine, Fleury Laboratory, S. Paulo, 1999.

Meadows, A. J. Scientific communication, Briquet de Lemos / Livros, Brasília, 1999.

Medical Professionalism Project. Medical professionalism in the new millenium: a physicians charter, The Lancet, vol. 359, February 9, 2002.

Millan, LR; De Marco, OLN; Rossi, E. E Arruda, PCV The psychological universe of the medical future / vocation, vicissitudes and perspectives, Casa do Psicólogo Livraria e Editora, S. Paulo, 1999.

Miller: Anesthesia, 5th Edition, Churchill Livingstone, New York, 2000.

Ministry of Health. Pandemic Influenza (H1N1) 2009, epidemiological report, year 1, nº 10, Nov. 2009.

Miroli, AB La Medicina en el Tiempo, Libreria El Ateneo, Buenos Aires, 1978.

Mlodinov, L. The drunk's walk - how chance determines our lives, Zahar, Rio de Janeiro, 2009.

Montgomery, R.; Conway, TW; Spector, AA, and Ginsberg, BH Biochemistry, a case-driven approach, 5th edition, Artes Médicas, S. Paulo, 1994.

Morabia, A. Snow and Farr: a scientic duet. Soz-Präventivmed, vol. 46: 217-224, 2001.

Moriyama, IM; Loy, RM; Robb-Smith, AHT History of the statistical classification of diseases and causes of death. Center for Disease Control and Prevention, Atlanta, 2011.

Moreira de Azevedo. The medical school of Rio de Janeiro, Historical news read at the Brazilian Historical and Geographic Institute, in 1866.

Morin. E. The seven knowledges necessary for the education of the future, 4th edition, Cortez Editora, S. Paulo, 2000.

Morral, J. Aristotle, Political Thought. University of Brasilia, Brasília, 1977.

Muss, HB Breast cancer and differential diagnosis of benign lesions. In Cecil Medicine, 23 rd ed., Elsevier Saunders, Philadelphia, 2008.

Nejar, C. History of Brazilian literature, Editora Leya, S. Paulo, 2011.

Nichols Jr., BL & Ballabriga, A., editors. History of Pediatrics (1850-1950), Raven Press, New York, 1991.

Nietzsche, N. Beyond good and evil, Editora Vozes, Petrópolis, 2009.

Novais, FA Approximations - History and Historiography Studies, Cosac Naify, S.Paulo, 2005.

Oda, AM; Piccinini, W.; Dalgalarrondo, P. Juliano Moreira (1873-1933): Founder of Scientific Psychiatry in Brazil, Am.J. Psychiatry 162: 4,666, 2005.

Oliveira, PM São Sebastião Hospital (1889-1905): a place for science and a lazaretto against epidemics. Dissertation (Master in Health Sciences), Casa de Oswaldo Cruz, FIOCRUZ, 2005.

Osório de Andrade, G. Morão, Rosa & Pimenta. News of the first three vernacular books on medicine in Brazil, State Public Archive of Pernambuco, Recife, 1956.

Padilha, PNA Nature and Art Rarities, Divided by the Four Elements, Francisco Luiz Ameno Patriarchal Workshop, Lisbon, 1759.

Page, TG, editor. Hippocrates, The Loeb Classical Library, Harvard University Press, London, 1957.

Papineau, D. Philosophy - Great thinkers, main foundations and schools of philosophy, Publifolha, S. Paulo, 2009.

Pan American Health Organization. EID Updates: Emerging and Reemerging Infectious Diseases, Region of the Americas. Dengue in Rio de Janeiro, Brazil, vol. 5, nº 9 (26 March 2008).

Perrenoud, P. Evaluation between two Logics, Artmed, Porto Alegre, 1999.

_____. Reflective practice in the profession of teacher: professionalization and pedagogical reason, Artmed, Porto Alegre, 2002.

Philippe, H. Les Premiers Soins et Secours D'urgence, Bourg Imprimerie du Journal, Paris, 1909.

Pinel, M. Abrégé des Transactions Philosophiques de La

Société Royale de Londres. Médecine et Chirurgie, Chez Buisson, Paris, 1791.

Pires, AST Evolution of the ideas of Physics, 2nd edition, Livraria da Física, S. Paulo, 2008.

Plato, Dialogues. Abril Cultural, S. Paulo, 1972.

Poland, GA et al. SARS-CoV-2 immunity: review and candidates of phase 3 vaccine candidates. Lancet 2020; 396: 1595-1606.

Porter, R. Medicina, the history of healing. Books & Books, Lisbon, 2002.

Powers, A. Diabetes mellitus. In Harrison's endocrinology, 16th ed., McGraw-Hill, New York, 2006.

Rapport, S. and Wright, H. Great adventures in medicine. The dial press, New York, 1961.

Reis Junior, A. The first to use anesthesia in surgery was not a dentist. It was the physician Crawford Williamson Long, Revista Brasileira de Anestesiologia; 56 (3): 304-324, 2006.

Ribeiro, L. Medicine in Colonial Brazil, Rio de Janeiro, 1971.

_____. Medicine in Brazil, National Press, Rio de Janeiro, 1940.

Robbins, FE Tetrabiblos, Book Three: of bodily injuries and diseases. Harvard University Press, 1940.

Rocha, L A. Annaes of Pernambuco medicine (1842-1844), Pernambuco Department of Education and Culture, Recife, 1977.

Root-Bernstein, R. and Root-Bernstein, M. The incredible history of medicines, Editora Campus Ltda., Rio de Janeiro, 1998.

Roberts, JM History of the World, 3rd edition, Ediouro, Rio de Janeiro, 2001.

Rosen, G. A History of Public Health, 2nd Edition, Editora UNESP, S. Paulo, 1994.

Russel, B. History of Western Philosophy, 3 volumes, Companhia Editora Nacional, S. Paulo, 1957.

_____. History of Western Thought, Ediouro Publications S. A., Rio de Janeiro, 2001.

Safranski, R. Heidegger, a master between good and evil, Geração Editorial, S. Paulo, 2000.

Santos Filho, L. General history of Brazilian medicine, 2 vols., Hucitec, S. Paulo, 1977.

_____. Short history of Brazilian medicine, S.Paulo Editora SA, S. Paulo, 1966.

Santos, RV and Coimbra Jr., CEA., Organizers. Health & Indigenous Peoples, Editora Fiocruz, Rio de Janeiro, 1994.

Sasson, D. Mona Lisa - the history of the most famous painting in the world, Editora Record, Rio de Janeiro, 2004.

Scliar, M. The transformed passion. History of medicine in literature. Companhia das Letras, S. Paulo, 1996.

Scliar, M. and Chagas Filho, C. Médicos, HC-FMUSP, special edition, year 1, nº 5, December 1998.

Self, WH et al. Effect of hydroxychloroquine on clinical status at 14 days in hospitalized patients with COVID-19. JAMA 2020; 22240: 1-11.

Senet, A. Man discovers his body (the novel of physiology).Editora Itatiaia Ltda., Belo Horizonte, 1958.

Segre, M. and Cohen, C. Bioética, 2nd edition, Edusp, 1999.

Shipley, AE editor. Lectures on the history of physiology, Cambridge University Press, Cambridge, 1901.

Schopenhauer, A. The Wisdom of Life, Golden Books, S. Paulo, 2007.

Silva, MRB; Ferla, Le Gallian, DMC A "library without walls": history of the creation of BIREME. History, Sciences, Health - Manguinhos, Rio de Janeiro, Vol. 13 (1): 91-112, 2006.

Silvers, RB, organizer. Forgotten stories of science, Peace and Earth, S. Paulo, 1997.

Simmons, J. The 100 greatest scientists in history, Editora Bertrand do Brasil, Rio de Janeiro, 2002.

Simmons, JG Médicos & Descobridores, Lives that created today's medicine, Editora Record, Rio de Janeiro, 2004.

Singer, C. A brief history of anatomy and physiology from the Greeks to Harvey, Editora da Unicamp, Campinas, 1996.

_____. Science, Medicine and History, 2 vols., Oxford University Press, London, 1953.

Smith, A. The wealth of nations, research on its nature and causes, Abril SA, S. Paulo, 1983.

Smith, D. Philosophy professor wants to resurrect Freud. http://www.uol.com.br/times/nytimes. Accessed on November 4, 2000.

Sournia, JC History of Medicine, Piaget Institute, Lisbon, 1996.

Sousa, G. History of Portuguese medicine during the expansion, Themes and Debates - Círculo de Autores, Lisbon, 2013.

Snow, J. On the mode of communication of cholera, London, 1855.

Starobinski, J. History of Medicine, Livraria Morais Editora, Lisbon, 1967.

Stuart-Harris, CH; Schild, GC Influenza, the viruses and the disease, Edward Arnold Ltd., London, 1976.

Sevcemko, N. The vaccine revolt - insane minds in rebel bodies, Brasiliense, S. Paulo, 1984.

Sharma, BK Contribution of astrology in medicine. Bulletin of the Indian Institute of History of Medicine, vol. 37 (1): 45-62, 2007.

Silveira, AJT Medicine and Spanish Influenza of 1918, Tempo, Rio de Janeiro; nº 19: 91-105, 2005.

Tang, W. and Eisenbrand, G. Chinese drugs of plant origin, Springer-Verlag, Berlin, 1992.

Thorwald, J. The century of surgeons, Hemus Editora Ltda., S. Paulo, 1998.

_____. The secret of the old doctors, Melhoramentos, S.Paulo, 1962.

Toynbee, A. A Study of History, 2nd edition, Editora Universidade de Brasília, Brasília, 1987.

Vasconcelos, I. Asclepius historian, Brazilian Institute of Medical History, Rio de Janeiro, 1964.

Vieira, S. and Hossne, WS Ethics and scientific methodology, Pioneira, S. Paulo, 1998.

Volcy, C. History of the concept of cause and sickness: parallelism between medicine and plant pathology. Iatreia, vol.20 (4): 407-421, 2007.

Walther, IF Masterpieces of Western painting, Taschen, Köln, 2002.

Weatherford, J. The History of Money. Editora Business, 1999.

Weber, M. Protestant ethics and the spirit of capitalism, 4th edition, Livraria Pioneira Editora, S. Paulo, 1947.

White, M. Leonardo, the first scientist, Editora Record, Rio de Janeiro, 2002.

Wynder, EL and Graham, EA Tobacco smoking as a possible etiologic factor in bro n chiogenic carcinoma. JAMA, vol. 143 (4): 329-336, 1950.

[1] Shakespeare, W. Complete work, vol. I, José Aguilar Editora, Rio de Janeiro, 1969.

[2] *Approaches, History Studies and Historiography*.

[3] *Sources for the history of health sciences in Brazil (1808-1930)*.

[4] Quoted by Richard Leonardo, in *History of Medical Thought*. The word philosophy means, in Greek, love of wisdom.

[5] Johannes Hessen, *Theory of knowledge*.

[6] *Philosophy of History*.

[7] In The Lost Art of Healing.

[8] In *The seven knowledge necessary for the education of the future*.

[9] With a student-centered teaching methodology, interactive pedagogy and an eminently formative assessment.

[10] Idea shared with Hannah Arendt.

[11] Including injuries and deaths in traffic accidents, homicides and suicides.

[12] Quoted by Simmons in *The 100 Greatest Scientists in History*.

[13] Quoted by Jean-Claude Guillebaud, in *The Force of Conviction*.

[14] In *History of Medicine*.

[15] In *The structure of scientific revolutions*.

[16]

Ambrogio Donini, in *Brief History of Religions*.

[17] Greek historian who lived in the 5th century BC

[18] In *Heroes of History*.

[19]

According to Singer, in *Science, Medicine and History*.

[20] In *A history of medicine*.

[21] According to Hegel, in *Philosophy of History.*

[22]

Ambrogio Donini, in *Brief History of Religions*.

[23] According to Berlingoff and Gouvea, in *Mathematics through the Times*.

[24] Bertrand Russel on Pythagoras: "I don't know of any man

who has been so influential in the sphere of thought."

[25] Aristotle believed that the characteristics of each species were fixed, with no possibility of evolution among living beings.

[26] The Empedocles Theory of Agrigento, who lived in the first half of the 5th century BC

[27] On the art of medicine.

[28] In *Philosophy of History*.

[29] Lopes, in *Medicine in Time*.

[30] Christianity was declared an official religion in the year 391, according to Guillebaud.

[31]

Durant, in *Heroes of History*.

[32] In *The History of Money*.

[33] Singer C. Science, Medicine and History, 2 vols., Oxford University Press, London, 1953.

[34] Sharma, BK Contribution of astrology in medicine. Bulletin of the Indian Institute of History of Medicine, vol. 37 (1): 45-62, 2007.

[35] Machado, C. A. The role of translation in the transmission of science: the case of Ptolemy's Tetrabiblos. Thesis for obtaining the title of Doctor of Letters at PUC-Rio, Rio de Janeiro, 273 p., 2010.

[36] Robbins, FE Tetrabiblos. Book Three: of bodily injuries and diseases, Harvard University Press, 1940.

[37] Volcy, C. History of cause and sick concepts: parallelism between medicine and phytopathology. Iatreia, vol.20 (4): 407-421, 2007.

[38] In Material Civilization, Economics and Capitalism: 15th-18th centuries. Cotian structures.

[39] In *A brief history of Brazil*.

[40] Op. Cit.

[41] Luís de Camões, *Os Lusíadas*, Canto V.

[42] Calder, R. *Man and medicine*.

[43] According to Sournia, what would have happened was poisoning by a parasitic rye mushroom (ergotism), which reaching small arteries of the limbs would cause considerable pain and burning, followed by spontaneous amputations.

[44] *Republic*, by Plato.

[45] Set of concepts about man, nature and knowledge itself that allow the development of tools that lead to the continuous construction of scientific knowledge.

[46] The inventor of the telescope was the Dutchman Hans Lippershey, in 1608.

[47] As in the *Dialogue, due to the massimi sistemi dei mondo - Tolemaic and Copernican,* he justifies his support for Copernicus' theory.

[48] In *Leonardo, the first scientist*.

[49] Koestler, A. in *The Man and the Universe*.

[50] According to Brody, the first scientific society appeared in Italy, in 1657, under the name of Experimentation Academy.

[51] According to Durant, in *Nova Atlântida*, Bacon guided the objectives of this scientific society.

[52] Calder, R. Op. Cit.

[53] The creation of the Society of Jesus was the most effective reaction of the Catholic Church to the Protestant reform, with the intention of facing up to the Protestant schools through a powerful pedagogical-educational action.

[54] In Pajé: reconstruction and survival.

[55] Ceremonial chief, priest, prophet, diviner, healer, blesser and sorcerer.

[56] In *To understand science.*

[57] In *The Social Contract.*

[58] According to Foucault, in *The Birth of the Clinic*, cited by Roy Porter.

[59] In *History of Madness*.

[60] That is, from feudalism, where the basis of the economy was the land, to capitalism where the production of goods, on a large scale, happens in factories, instead of artisanal production, as before.

[61] Max Weber, in *Protestant ethics and the spirit of capitalism*.

[62] In Material Civilization, economics and capitalism: 15th-18th centuries, The time of the world.

[63] With working hours of up to 16 hours a day, employing children and with poor working conditions.

[64] In *Forgotten Stories of Science*.

[65] Ibid.

[66] Hardy, A. Water and the search for public health in London in the eighteen and nineteen centuries. Medical History, vol. 28 (3): 250-282, 1984.

[67] Ibid.

[68] Ibid.

[69] Cerda, JL and Valdivia, GC John Snow, the cholera epidemic and the birth of clinical epidemiology, Revista Chilena de Infectologia, 24 (4): 331-334, 2007.

[70] Miasms could be defined as any source considered harmful, which would corrupt the air and attack our organism. Thus epidemic outbreaks of infectious diseases would be caused by the pernicious state of the atmosphere.

[71] Snow, J. On the mode of communication of cholera, London, 1849.

[72] Moriyama, IM; Loy, RM; Robb-Smith, AHT History of the statistical classification of diseases and causes of death, Center for Disease Control and Prevention, Atlanta, 2011.

[73] Bingham, P.; Verlander, NQ; Cheal, MJ John Snow, William Farr and the 1849 outbreak of cholera that affected London: a re working of the data highlights the importance of the water supply, Public Health 118: 387-394, 2004.

[74] Eyler, JM The changing assessments of John Snow's and William Farr's cholera studies, Soz - Pr äventivmed, 46: 225-232, 2001.

[75] Morabia, A. Snow and Farr: a scientific duet, Soz - Pr äventivmed, 46: 217-224, 2001.

[76]

Cited by Johannes Hessen, in *Theory of knowledge*.

[77] Max Schoen, according to Leonardo, in *History of Medical Thought*.

[78] Quoted by Antonio Damásio in *O Descartes' Error*.

[79] Considered by John Maynard Keynes to be the first economist in history.

[80] Kevin Davies, in *Deciphering the genome*.

[81] He published the book *Pathologische Untersuchungen*, in 1840, where he reformulated the ideas of his predecessors.

[82] Thorwald, in *The Century of Surgeons.*

[83] Only with the introduction of antibiotics, after the discovery of penicillin, was the infection overcome.

[84] Oda, A. M.; Piccini, W.; Dalgalarrondo, P. Juliano Moreira: Founder of Scientific Psychiatry in Brazil. Am. J. Psychiatry 162: 4, April 2005.

[85]

In *The Neurosciences*, Rockefeller University Press, 1970.

[86] Freud, in *A difficulty in the path of psychoanalysis*.

[87] Habermas, a contemporary German philosopher, considers Psychoanalysis the paradigm of a critical science, which works by dissolving pathological structures that inhibit the subject's free communication with himself and with others.

[88] According to Magnoli, in *A drop of blood*.

[89]

Doctrine of Gnosticism, cited by John G. Gunnel, in *Political Theory*.

[90] Mahmood, SS et al. The Framingham heart study and the epidemiology of cardiovascular diseases: a historical perspective. Lancet, 383 (9921): 999-1008, 2014.

[91] Dawber, T.; Meadors, G and Moore Jr., F. Epidemiological approaches to heart disease: The Framingham sudy, American Journal of Public Health, vol. 41: 279-286, 1951.

[92] Bonita, R.; Beaglehole, R. and Kjellström, T. Basic Epidemiology, 2nd edition, World Health Organization, Livraria Santos Editora, S. Paulo, 2010.

[93] Fox, CS et al. Temporal trends in coronary heart disease mortality and sudden cardiac death from 1950 to 1999: the Framjngham heart study. Circulation, 110: 522-527, 2004.

[94] Duncan, BB et al. Chronic non-communicable diseases in Brazil: priority for coping and research. Revista de Saúde Pública, 46 (Supl.): 126-134, 2012.

[95] Doll, R. and Hill, The. B. Smoking and carcinoma of the lung. British Medical Journal, 2 (4682): 739-748, 1950.

[96] Wynder, E. L. and Graham, EA Tobacco smoking as a pos-

sible etiologic factor in brochiogenic carcinoma. JAMA, 143 (4): 329-336, 1950.

[97] Alberg, AJ; Shopland, D. R, and Cummings, KM The 2014 Surgeon General's Report: Commemorating the 50th Anniversary of the Report of the Advisory Committee to the US Surgeon General and Updating the Evidence on the Health Consequences of Cigarette Smoking. American journal of Epidemiology, 179 (4): 403-412, 2014.

[98] Hirayama, T. Non-smoking wives f heavy smokers have a higher risk of lung cancer. British Medical Journal, 282 (6259): 183-185, 1981.

[99] Alberg, AJ Op. C it.

[100]

Several species of plants belong to euphorbiates. In Brazil, the rubber tree is one of the most important.

[101] In recent years there has been a drop in infant mortality rates, mainly due to the actions of community agents from the Family Health program and non-governmental organizations such as Pastoral da Criança, an organization that monitors 1.6 million children and more 70,000 pregnant women in more than 32,000 communities across the country.

[102] According to Laura Camargo M. Feeuerwerker, in *Changes in medical education and medical residency in Brazil.*

[103] Tribuna especial, Physician up to date, Medical Association of Brasília, n.154, March-April 2014.

www.ingramcontent.com/pod-product-compliance
Lightning Source LLC
Chambersburg PA
CBHW072027230526
45466CB00020B/949